Roberto Patarca-Montero, MD, PhD

Treatment of Chronic Fatigue Syndrome in the Antiviral Revolution Era

Pre-publication
REVIEWS,
COMMENTARIES,
EVALUATIONS . . .

"**A** fascinating walking tour through the history of antibiosis, genomics, AIDS, and then CFS. Sections on the development of anti-infectives from research on HIV are succinct and elucidating, but I am most intrigued by Patarca-Montero's explanation of the immune system in CFS and his step-by-step approach to immunological and antiviral therapies.

I don't know how Patarca does it! He has the uncanny ability to take very complicated and diverse subjects and make easy reading out of them. Interesting reading and a great reference."

Charles W. Lapp, MD
Director, Hunter-Hopkins Center, Charlotte, NC;
Assistant Consulting Professor, Division of Community and Family Medicine, Duke University

"**T**his book is a remarkable treatise relating to the scientific exercises of a number of devoted and highly experienced experts in the developing areas of genomics and viruses and the interrelationship that is developing as specific treatment for viral diseases increases. Professor Patarca-Montero is extremely wise in the way he summates all the varying pharmacological approaches without suggesting that any magic bullet has yet been found. In a very extensive survey he has, however, shown a balanced appreciation for the varying avenues that have been explored in efforts to produce remedial results. As the author remarks, `The ultimate proof of a therapeutic concept is of course found only in the clinic or at the bedside.' This is an excellent book for all medical professionals."

Dr. John Richardson, MB, BS
Newcastle Research Group, UK;
Author, *Enteroviral and Toxin Mediated Encephalomyelitis/ Chronic Fatigue Syndrome and Other Organ Pathologies*

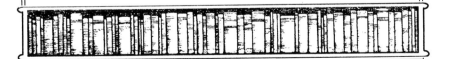

More pre-publication
REVIEWS, COMMENTARIES, EVALUATIONS . . .

"**A** must-have manual of antiviral drug therapy for innovative physicians and their CFS patients. Professor Patarca-Montero's scholarly and extensively referenced assessment of the CFS antiviral drug revolution provides a promising new alternative choice for patients."

R. Bruce Duncan, FRCS, FRACS, FAAOA
Director, Virutherapy Clinic,
Wellington, New Zealand;
Author, *CFIDS, Fibromyalgia,
and the Virus-Allergy Link*

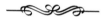

"**T**his book is well written, informative, and a must-read for CFS physicians. It is comprehensive and provides an excellent historic account of microbial agents and antimicrobial therapies and transfer factors that have

been utilized to treat CFS patients with some degree of success. Since CFS etiology is still being investigated, the book describes the viral agents that have been implicated in the pathogenesis of CFS. The beauty of the book is that it reviews various studies without making any favorable or adverse remarks, thus allowing readers to judge for themselves.

Even though it is designed to reach CFS physicians and researchers, CFS patients may benefit from knowing what types of therapies have been attempted to combat CFS. There are many references, so readers can seek more details if necessary. This book is a good reference for medical libraries."

Dharam V. Ablashi, DVM, MS, Dip. Bact.
Director,
Herpesvirus Programs,
Advanced Biotechnologies, Inc.,
Columbia, Maryland

The Haworth Medical Press®
An Imprint of The Haworth Press, Inc.
New York • London • Oxford

Treatment of Chronic Fatigue Syndrome in the Antiviral Revolution Era

THE HAWORTH MEDICAL PRESS®
Chronic Fatigue Syndrome, Fibromyalgia Syndrome, and Myalgic Encephalomyelitis

Roberto Patarca-Montero, MD, PhD
Senior Editor

Concise Encyclopedia of Chronic Fatigue Syndrome by Roberto Patarca-Montero

CFIDS, Fibromyalgia, and the Virus-Allergy Link: Hidden Viruses, Allergies, and Uncommon Fatigue/Pain Disorders by R. Bruce Duncan

Phytotherapy of Chronic Fatigue Syndrome: Evidence-Based and Potentially Useful Botanicals in the Treatment of CFS by Roberto Patarca-Montero

Concise Encyclopedia of Fibromyalgia and Myofacial Pain by Roberto Patarca-Montero

Treatment of Chronic Fatigue in the Antiviral Revolution Era by Roberto Patarca-Montero

Chronic Fatigue Syndrome, Christianity, and Culture: Between God and an Illness by James M. Rotholz

Treatment of Chronic Fatigue Syndrome in the Antiviral Revolution Era

Roberto Patarca-Montero, MD, PhD

The Haworth Medical Press®
An Imprint of The Haworth Press, Inc.
New York   London   Oxford

Published by

The Haworth Medical Press®, an imprint of The Haworth Press, Inc., 10 Alice Street, Binghamton, NY 13904-1580

Medicine is an ever-changing science. As new research and clinical experience broaden our knowledge, changes in treatment and drug therapy are required. While many suggestions for drug usages are made herein, the book is intended for educational purposes only, and the author, editor, and publisher do not accept liability in the event of negative consequences incurred as a result of information presented in this book. We do not claim that this information is necessarily accurate by the rigid, scientific standard applied for medical proof, and therefore make no warranty, expressed or implied, with respect to the material herein contained. Therefore the patient is urged to check the product information sheet included in the package of each drug he or she plans to administer to be certain the protocol followed is not in conflict with the manufacturer's inserts. When a discrepancy arises between these inserts and information in this book, the physician is encouraged to use his or her best professional judgment.

The author has exhaustively researched all available sources to ensure the accuracy and completeness of the information contained in this book. The publisher and author assume no responsibility for errors, inaccuracies, omissions, or any inconsistency herein.

Cover design by Marylouise E. Doyle.

Library of Congress Cataloging-in-Publication Data

Patarca-Montero, Roberto
    Treatment of chronic fatigue syndrome in the antiviral revolution era / Roberto Patarca-Montero.
      p. ; cm.
    Includes bibliographical references and index.
    ISBN 0-7890-1253-7 (hard : alk. paper) — ISBN-0-7890-1254-5 (soft : alk paper)
    1. Chronic fatigue syndrome. 2. Antiviral agents. I. Title.
[DNLM: 1. Fatigue Syndrome, Chronic—drug therapy. 2. Antiviral Agents—therapeutic use. WC 500 P294t 2001]
    RB150.F37 P386 2001
    616'.0478—dc21
                                                                2001016939

CONTENTS

ABOUT THE AUTHOR

Roberto Patarca-Montero, MD, PhD, HCLD, is Assistant Professor of Medicine, Microbiology, and Immunology and also serves as Research Director of the E. M. Papper Laboratory of Clinical Immunology at the University of Miami School of Medicine. Previously, he was Assistant Professor of Pathology at the Dana-Farber Cancer Institute and Harvard Medical School in Boston. Dr. Patarca-Montero serves as editor of *Critical Reviews in Oncogenesis* and the *Journal of Chronic Fatigue Syndrome.* He is also the author or co-author or more than 100 articles in journals or books, including *The Concise Encyclopedia of Chronic Fatigue Syndrome* (Haworth, 2000). He is currently conducting research on immunotherapy of AIDS and chronic fatigue syndrome. Dr. Patarca-Montero is a member of the Board of Directors of the American Association for Chronic Fatigue Syndrome and the Acquired Non-HIV Immune Diseases Foundation.

Preface

The growing rate of discovery and use of antiviral agents, the first fruits of the expanding genomics revolution, brightens the start of the millennium. Throughout most of the past century, physicians could offer patients no treatments for infections caused by viruses, entities that commandeer the biosynthetic apparatus of a host cell to reproduce. Prevention of infection, by vaccination campaigns and other public health measures, was the approach that eliminated smallpox worldwide by 1980, and seems likely soon to eliminate polio.

Viral scourges continue to exact a huge toll.[1] The disastrous AIDS pandemic is merely the most well known. Complications of hepatitis B and C kill approximately one million people each year, and measles continues to be the cause of deaths among children even though effective vaccines exist for measles and hepatitis B. Rotavirus, which causes diarrhea, takes the lives of hundreds of thousands, mainly children. Other viral diseases seem to be restricted to specific areas. Ross River virus disease causes acute illness in parts of Australia, and the deadly Ebola and hantavirus occasionally emerge to wreak bloody havoc in Africa and the American south. West Nile virus is terrorizing New York and is responsible for several deaths. Many mysterious historical outbreaks of disease were probably viral, among them Tapanui flu, which sickened thousands of people in New Zealand in the 1970s, and Akureyri disease, which affected 1,000 people in a small town in Iceland in 1948 and 1949.

Some innovative scientists have proposed, even as early as a century ago, that a much wider range of illnesses than is generally thought might actually be caused by viruses. These scientists have challenged conventional medical wisdom to expand the realm of diseases of possible viral etiology to include pathological processes as diverse as atherosclerosis [2-9] and autoimmune disease.[10-24]

This book addresses the scientific rationale, historical evolution, clinical trials, and lines of research on the use of antiviral agents for the treatment of chronic fatigue syndrome (CFS), a disease entity that has been postulated to be of viral or autoimmune etiology. Although none of the therapeutic approaches covered in this book has proven to be universally effective and their inclusion does not represent an endorsement by the author, antiviral therapy may prove to have a role in controlling at least some of the symptomatology associated with CFS. The approaches include the use of synthetic small molecule drugs, herbal products, vaccines, and other substances and interventions that directly interfere with virus infection, indirectly help fight them by boosting the immunological defense system, or help correct the imbalances in the immune system that are left as their sequel. It is the hope of the author that this compendium extracted from the biomedical literature, published patent filings, and private company announcements on their unpublished research will serve as a useful reference guide for health care professionals and patients alike.

Chapter 1

The Antiviral Era

The dawn of this century is brightened by the growing frequency of use and discovery of antiviral agents, the first fruits of the expanding genomics revolution. This new antiviral era, which flourished from the knowledge provided by the molecular biological characterization of the genetic makeup of viruses, is engendering new chemical and biological agents that are able to treat and not just prevent viral diseases. Hypotheses have also been rekindled that challenge conventional wisdom to expand the realm of diseases of viral etiology to include pathological processes, such as atherosclerosis and autoimmune disease, that would not have been previously thought as secondary to infectious processes. Regardless of whether the latter hypotheses prove to be correct, the experience that is being garnered in this antiviral revolution also serves, in the light of the information now available on the genetic makeup of human beings, as an encouraging paradigm for the development of drugs to treat all kinds of human diseases.

One of the diseases of possible viral origin that started to receive close attention in the latter part of the twentieth century is chronic fatigue syndrome. Chronic fatigue syndrome (CFS) is characterized by debilitating fatigue that is not attributable to known clinical conditions, has lasted for more than six months, has reduced the activity level of a previously healthy person by more than 50 percent, and has been accompanied by flu-like symptoms (e.g., pharyngitis, adenopathy, low-grade fever, myalgia, arthralgia, headache), and neuropsychological manifestations (e.g., difficulty concentrating, exercise intolerance, and sleep disturbances).[25-31]

Although syndromes are clusters of nonchance associations, and the components of a syndrome can be generally related to a common element, the cause of CFS still remains to be determined. CFS is frequently of a sudden onset. Possible precipitating factors include infections, psychiatric trauma, and exposure to toxins.[31-34] Even among those who favor a viral etiology for CFS, it is not yet clear whether CFS is a consequence of a chronic viral infection or an acute viral infection which resolves but whose sequel in the form of autoimmunity or other manifestations is responsible for the pathology seen. As detailed in Chapter 2, many families of viruses have been studied in association with CFS, including herpesviruses, enteroviruses, retroviruses, lentiviruses, adeno-viruses, Borna disease virus, parvoviruses, and arboviruses. It has also been proposed that reactivation of certain viruses may play a role in the pathophysiology of CFS but may not be its primary cause.

Based on the postulates of viral and autoimmune etiologies of CFS, several interventions have been designed and tested and are covered in the following chapters. These interventions have become possible because of the growing armamentarium of antiviral agents in molecular medicine and their widespread use in clinical practice—changes which have, in turn, arisen thanks to a confluence of novel approaches and a fresh look at past clinical wisdom. It is therefore instructive to review the historical background of the current developments in antiviral therapy.

The current antiviral drug revolution can trace its first roots to the contributions of scientists such as Spallanzani, who compellingly challenged the theory of spontaneous generation supported by the Roman Catholic Church and revealed the existence of a biological microcosm invisible to the naked eye that could account for many occurrences that were until then shrouded by a cloud of mystical religious beliefs; from the growth of mold on a wet surface to the transmission of certain diseases. Although Girolamo Fracastoro taught, in 1530, that syphilis was a contagious disease spread by "seeds," and in 1683 Antony van Leeuwenhoek observed bacteria by using a crude microscope, it was the nineteenth century, with the contributions of scientists such as Louis Pasteur and Robert Koch, that saw the consolidation of the germ theory of disease and the flourishing of microbiology thanks to the definitive isolation of infectious organisms and the demonstration of their association with disease.[35] Around that time, Dmitri Ivanowski and Martinus Beijerinck described viruses as small infectious agents that could pass through bacteria-stopping filters. Following the identification of infectious organisms, immunology was born as a discipline aimed at unraveling the mechanisms used by the body to control and defeat them. Shortly thereafter, modern infectious disease medicine was inaugurated with the discovery of antibiotics in the early part of the twentieth century, an accomplishment that was based on the observation that fungi produced substances that were able to kill bacteria. The isolation and medical use of penicillin and other naturally occurring antibiotics, as well as the development of their synthetic derivatives, has allowed to control the spread and severity of bacterial infections and to preclude the reemergence of vast bacterial epidemics, such as the bubonic plague caused by the bacteria *Yersinia pestis* that killed a large portion of the human population in the Middle Ages.

Unlike the case with bacteria, viruses have no known natural enemies from which to isolate antibiotic-like substances, and, until the mid-1980s, viral infections were thought to be inherently preventable in some cases but generally untreatable. Many viral epidemics, such as polio, yellow fever, whooping cough, AIDS, and viral hepatitis, have received worldwide attention in the past and during this century. There are also many historical accounts of diseases of presumed viral etiology that present similar to CFS, including George Reinhold Forster's description of the Tapanui flu and the documentation of Akureyri or Iceland disease.[36,37] The first half of the twentieth century witnessed the first successful approach to control the spread of several viral infections: the development and worldwide use of vaccines. The concept of vaccination was originally developed by Jenner in eighteenth-century England based on the observation that milkmaids exposed to cows with cowpox were protected from smallpox. In this case, a subclinical infection with one virus was protective of an infection with a related one. The latter concept was also extended to the treatment of various infectious diseases by giving the patient even unrelated but more innocuous infectious diseases. Although in many cases the treatment was worse than the disease, the therapeutic approach was somehow useful with particular combinations of infectious agents.

Outstanding triumphs of worldwide vaccination programs have been the eradication of smallpox and predictably soon of poliomyelitis.[38] After smallpox was eliminated as an infectious disease in Great Britain in 1962, two outbreaks occurred, one in 1973 and one in 1978, when smallpox virus under study in laboratories infected susceptible individuals. In both incidents, deaths resulted.[38] With the eradication of poliomyelitis throughout the world soon to be accomplished, steps are being taken to prevent polioviruses that remain in laboratories from escaping into the community and causing disease. These examples stress the need for universal availability of vaccines to effectively eradicate the diseases they cause. Unfortunately, we do not have vaccines against all viruses; even in the cases for which we do have vaccines, the vaccine is not universally available. The dramatic success in immunizing children against childhood diseases stands in stark contrast to the much lower percentages of adults who are adequately immunized against common adult diseases. In the case of the flu vaccine, the influenza virus keeps changing, the vaccine has to be updated every year, and it is therefore not fully protective against all viral strains.

One alternative to vaccines has been the use of injections of immunoglobulins, the natural bullets that the body produces to kill foreign invaders. Not too long ago, physicians advocated the use of immunoglobulin injections as a way to "boost" the body's immune defenses and heighten resistance against microbes. The latter reasoning was perhaps again reflective of the old wisdom of using one infection to protect against another with the added refinement of using the natural mediators of the body's attack machinery against infections instead of the infectious agent itself.

The limitations of antibodies as antiviral therapeutic agents still leave us with having to treat viral infections and, unlike the case with bacteria, we do not know the natural enemies of viruses from which to isolate antibiotic-like substances. The Nobel laureate Paul Ehrlich preached in the early twentieth century about the usefulness of discovering chemical substances that would act as "magic bullets" against infectious agents with little or no untoward effects to humans. Although the "magic bullets" studied in Ehrlich's days were too toxic, Ehrlich's vision inspired the pharmaceutical industry's search for therapeutic small molecules, a task that has now been rekindled with the help of modern biology.

Viruses were the first microorganisms whose complete genetic makeup was characterized. The information on viral genes and their protein products has allowed to develop a series of chemicals with targeted antiviral activity. The advent of the acquired immunodeficiency syndrome (AIDS) pandemic in the second half of the twentieth century became the largest challenge to infectious disease medicine of the modern era. The discovery and characterization of the first human pathogenic retrovirus, the human T-cell leukemia/lymphoma virus type I (HTLV-I),[39-42] facilitated the discovery of the etiological agent of AIDS, the human immunodeficiency virus type 1 (HIV-1). Determination of the primary structure of HIV-1, first known as HTLV-III or LAV (lymphadenopathy virus) and computerized analysis of the amino acid sequence of the gene products it encodes provided the targets and, at the same time, the reagents to develop rapid and sensitive assay systems for testing potential therapeutic agents with anti-HIV activity.[43-45] Therefore, anti-HIV therapeutic medicines were born from the marriage between molecular and cellular biology, traditional therapeutic small molecule screening, and the then-incipient discipline of bioinformatics,[46-62] a marriage that also fueled the vigorous resurgence of genomics research.

The first databases of nucleic acid and protein sequences were created in the late 1970s. The computerization of algorithms for primary structure comparisons and secondary structure predictions (hydrophilicity and folding structures) and their use to analyze the genetic makeup of the AIDS virus in the framework of the knowledge garnered over decades for other known viruses quickly provided the targets for the development of anti-HIV agents. It is therefore the case that, although nonprimate viruses were the first microorganisms whose complete genetic makeup was characterized, it was not until the complete sequence of the AIDS virus became available in an unprecedented record time thanks in part to the strong public pressure for basic and clinical research that the information on viral genes·and their protein products triggered an exponential growth in the development of chemicals with targeted antiviral activity.

Before the AIDS epidemic, the only antiviral agent that had been widely introduced to clinical practice with modest acceptance was acyclovir. The drug acyclovir, which is used to treat infections by herpes simplex viruses, the causative agents of the most feared viral venereal disease before the AIDS era, inhibits the viral DNA polymerase, a protein that is needed for the virus to replicate. The drug, after chemical modification by the body, affects mainly the viral DNA polymerase because the latter is sufficiently different from its human cell counterpart. Similar in concept to acyclovir, the first medication introduced for AIDS and diseases related to HIV-1 infection was 3'-azido-2', 3'-dideoxythymidine (formerly known as azidothymidine [AZT] and currently known as zidovudine [ZDV]), a nucleoside analog that inhibits reverse transcriptase, a critical enzyme for the replication of HIV.[56-62] It is noteworthy that the discovery of reverse transcriptase several decades before the characterization of the AIDS virus had demolished the dogma in molecular biology that genetic information could flow only from DNA to RNA to protein by demonstrating that information could also flow from RNA to DNA, as was exemplified by the life cycle of retroviruses.

The initial success of AZT opened the door for the development of other antiretroviral agents, and no doubt exists today that antiretroviral chemotherapy can bring about reduction of viral load and clinical benefits to HIV-infected individuals. Besides AZT, a variety of 2',3'-dideoxynucleosides have been added to the anti-HIV armamentarium, among them ddI or didanosine, ddC or zalcitabine, d4T or stavudine, and 3TC or lamivudine. Many more are undergoing clinical or preclinical testing. Nonnucleoside reverse transcriptase inhibitors, including nevirapine and delavirdine, have also become available and more will emerge in the near future. The high mutation rate of HIV has allowed the selection of viral strains resistant to antiretrovirals, a feature that has fed a constant need for new viral therapeutic targets. As the first clinical application of what has been termed pharmacogenomics, the genomics era has also provided the intermediate- and high-throughput tools to genotype AIDS virus strains from patients to determine their drug resistance patterns.

Changes in antiretroviral therapy choice based on the viral resistance patterns allow better control of viral load and disease progression.

A virus that has approximately 15 genes, such as HIV, presents a much more limited drug target repertoire than bacteria such as the gut-dwelling bacterium *Escherichia coli* with approximately 1,500 different proteins. The latter limitation in target variety has rendered the traditional random drug screening efforts for anti-HIV agents disappointing for the most part, a hurdle that has been the inspiration for the introduction of different drug development approaches. Approximately one decade after the introduction of AZT, the inhibitors of another viral enzyme, protease, were hailed on their way into clinics as the long-awaited panacea for AIDS. The viral protease is needed to cleave the original synthesis products of the virus to generate building blocks required for assembly of new viral particles. The successful development of HIV protease inhibitors is arguably the greatest achievement to date for the relatively new method of structure-based drug design.[63-67] The latter design is possible when the structure of the molecular target has been determined by X-ray crystallography, nuclear magnetic resonance (NMR), or remodeling. Unbeknown to many clinicians, the presence in the viral genome and the start point for the generation of the protease gene had been originally predicted in the early 1980s with accuracy down to one amino acid in the first round of analysis of the HIV sequence. But it was not until the structure of this enzyme was determined that the first design studies with HIV-1 began with HIV protease in the early 1990s. Many protease inhibitors are currently available on the market; saquinavir, ritonavir, indinavir, and nelfinavir, and another large group is in clinical and preclinical development.

The initial experience with anti-HIV therapy has evinced the greater efficacy, as compared to monotherapy, of appropriately combining multiple classes of antiviral agents in patients with HIV infection. As structure-based drug design methods improve, new therapeutic agents will be effectively developed against novel antiviral targets for HIV-1 therapy. The X-ray crystallography and NMR structures of several HIV-1-encoded proteins have been determined, including the reverse transcriptase, RNase H, integrase, matrix, capsid, nucleocapsid, Tat protein, and a domain of gp41. In addition, the structures of the cell surface proteins with which the envelope proteins of HIV interact have also been characterized; i.e., the envelope binding domains of CD4 and that of certain chemokine receptors, such as CCR5. The need to continue to search for and develop drugs against novel antiviral targets for HIV therapy should not be underestimated, because the prevalence of new drug-resistant variants of HIV that are insensitive to even the best current regimens of triple and quadruple combination therapy is rising at an alarming rate, especially in the context of patient nonadherence secondary to the complexity or financial burden of combined regimens.

The discovery of protease inhibitors also illustrates another important strength of the genomics approach to drug discovery. The characterization of the genetic makeup of HIV allowed to develop target-based screens to identify novel lead compounds for specific targets that would otherwise have gone unidentified in cell culture-based assays. In this respect, high-throughput protease assays were responsible for identifying nonpeptidic lead compounds that were subsequently developed into potent protease inhibitors with anti-HIV activity, even though the initial lead compounds had no measurable antiviral activity in tissue culture assays. Conversely, compounds that exhibit antiviral activity in a cell culture-based screen can now be subjected to a battery of mechanism-based tests to profile their mode of action.

The characterization of the genetic makeup of the AIDS virus is also helping to fine tune the development of AIDS vaccines aimed not only at triggering, as most conventional viral vaccines do, the production of antibodies, the natural bullets that cells of the body's immunological defense system produce to kill foreign invading agents, but also at stimulating the so-called cellular immunity, i.e., bringing into action other cells of the body's defense system that can directly kill the virus or the virus-infected cells. Again, in this front, the high mutation rate of the virus and the presence of different variants or clades of HIV in the major geographical areas affected by the epidemic has posed a formidable obstacle to the development of vaccines.[68]

The development of vaccines as well as the preclinical testing of drugs and therapeutic biologicals with anti-HIV activity have found a strong ally in the availability of several naturally derived or man-made animal models, most prominent among which are simian immunodeficiency virus (SIV)-infected macaques; mice with genetically determined severe combined immunodeficiency engrafted with human hematolymphoid cells from fetal liver, thymus, and lymph node (SCID-hu mice); and SCID mice reconstituted with human peripheral blood leukocytes (hu-PBL-SCID mice).[69,70] The search for and generation of appropriate animal models for drug and vaccine testing is crucial to the success of the genomics approach for the discovery of new pharmaceuticals and is proving to be a major bottleneck for the pharmaceutical industry.

In theory, antiviral drugs exert their effects by interacting with viral structural components, virally encoded enzymes, viral genomes, or specific host proteins such as cellular receptors, enzymes, or other factors required for viral replication. In principle, any virus-specific step in the viral replicative cycle that differs from that in normal host cell function can serve as a potential target for the development of antiviral therapy. The final litmus test of this approach to drug development takes place at the clinic or the bedside, a process that involves both demonstration of safety and efficacy of a medication, as well as a learning curve for the health care professional in the use of a new therapeutic agent or modality.

The battle against the AIDS virus, despite its limitations, has habituated clinicians to the concept of treating viral infections with drugs, and agents similar in concept to those used for the AIDS virus are now being aimed against the hepatitis viruses. Interestingly, the initial analysis of the HIV primary sequence and its comparison to that of other viruses also put in evidence the existence in hepatitis-B virus of a reverse transcriptase gene. Until then, the hepatitis-B virus had been believed to be a double-stranded DNA virus, and now it is known that, similar to retroviruses, it replicates through an RNA intermediate. Based on this realization, the nucleoside analog lamivudine is being used for the treatment of chronic hepatitis-B virus, while the nucleoside analog ribavirin (1-beta-D-ribofuranosyl-1,2,4-triazole-3-carboxamide) is part of the therapeutic arsenal for combating chronic infection with hepatitis C, an RNA virus. Ribavirin has also shown activity in vitro against dengue virus.[71]

The current use of nucleoside inhibitors extends to other viruses. For instance, ribavirin is the only drug available for treatment of respiratory syncytial virus infection, the leading cause of lower respiratory tract infection (pneumonia and bronchiolitis) in normal infants and children.[72] In the latter indication, ribavirin is delivered by a small particle aerosol generator and, to be effective, it must be started as early as possible. Although ribavirin aerosol has also been successfully used for the treatment of severe parainfluenza virus disease in some children with severe immunodeficiency, studies are thus far inadequate to establish efficacy. On the other hand, intravenous ribavirin has been used with successful responses in some cases of adenoviral infection. The latter experiences demonstrate another important area in the effective clinical use of the new drugs developed from the genomics revolution, namely their adequate delivery by several routes for different indications. In this respect, the genomics-based drug revolution has also fueled an exponential growth rate in the research on drug delivery systems, and many more innovative breakthroughs are on the horizon.

The influence of using antiviral agents to control HIV infection extends further to the battle against the flu.[73,74] Although two important proteins of influenza viruses were known for many years before the AIDS epidemic, it was not until recently that effective drugs that would target these enzymes were developed. Following the discovery in 1942 of an enzyme on the influenza virus surface that removed virus receptors from erythrocytes, the prediction was put forth that an inhibitor for said enzyme might be an effective antiviral agent. Although the first inhibitors of this viral enzyme known as neuraminidase were developed in 1969, it was not until 1993, after the crystal structure of the enzyme and improved understanding of the mechanism of catalysis had been achieved, that zanamivir was introduced as a potent and highly specific inhibitor of influenza neuraminidase activity. Inhaled zanamivir (Relenza; Glaxo Wellcome, Inc.) entered clinical trials in 1994 and is now licensed in Australia, Europe, and North America. The first orally active inhibitor, oseltamivir, was described in 1997. It has been approved in Switzerland, Canada, and the United States. A second oral agent entered clinical trials in 1999.

The influenza neuraminidase inhibitors represent a significant advance over the hemagglutinin inhibitors amantadine (Symmetrel; DuPont) and rimantadine (Flumadine; Forest Pharmaceuticals, Inc.) that were available for many years but rarely used in influenza therapy. Amantadine or rimantadine may be given orally early in the course for influenza type-A infections but are not effective for influenza type B. Ribavirin aerosol use has led to the reduction of symptoms in some patients with influenza, types A or B, infections. Amantadine, rimantadine, or zanamivir can also be used prophylactically in immunocompromised patients exposed to influenza-A virus infection. For those exposed to influenza B, only zanamivir is recommended, using one dose daily during the exposure period.[74] The neuraminidase as compared to the hemagglutinin inhibitors have a broader spectrum of antiviral activity (both influenza A and B as opposed to only A); less potential for emergence of clinically important resistance; better tolerability; and proven efficacy in reducing respiratory events leading to antibiotic use after influenza.

One alternative approach for prophylaxis of influenza and respiratory syncytial virus (RSV) infections has been the use of immunoglobulins, in particular preparations enriched in those directed specifically at particular viruses. RSV is the leading cause of lower respiratory tract infection (pneumonia and bronchiolitis) in normal infants and children. For example, seasonal prophylaxis of RSV infection, in the form of monthly infusions of RSV-polyclonal antibody or the injection of RSV humanized monoclonal antibody (palivizumab), has been effective in small infants with profound immunodeficiency, pulmonary compromise, and/or bone marrow transplant recipients. A series of antibodies against specific viral targets are being tested at the time and more will be developed as target display libraries continue to allow the selection of effective antibodies among samples with diversity in the thousands.

Many other antiviral agents are in the market and there are different categories of antiviral agents at various stages of drug development. For instance, the broad-spectrum capsid-binding agent pleconaril (VP 63843) shows promise for the treatment of rhinovirus infection, the virus causing the common cold, but the drug is available on a compassionate protocol use. Pleconaril may also have therapeutic efficacy in enteroviral aseptic meningoencephalitis. An antiviral drug that could hardly have been conceived of before the advent of genomics is based on the principle of "antisense": the drug, fomivirsen, consists of nucleic acid sequences that bind to and neutralize a crucial component of the reproducing virus. It is approved in the United States for the treatment of cytomegalovirus retinis. One drug being tested in patients with hepatitis C consists of a ribozyme: an RNA molecule that cuts specific viral RNA sequences.

Besides the traditional viral infections, the antiviral agents being developed may also help in the control of diseases where the body loses its balanced control of internal processes. For instance, some viruses have become part of our genetic makeup, the so-called endogenous viruses, and their expression serves some functions that are being unraveled. The body appears to keep the expression of endogenous viruses in check, and it has been noted that the unregulated expression of endogenous viruses may play a role in some autoimmune diseases, maladies in which the body attacks itself by making antibodies against its own tissues. One example of such a disease is Sjoegren's syndrome, a malady in which the body makes antibodies against the salivary and lacrimal glands and the person suffers dry eyes and mouth. Overexpression of the endogenous viruses called intracisternal A particles have been associated with Sjoegren's syndrome.

The realm of antiviral therapy may soon extend to diseases that are not traditionally thought of as viral in origin. For instance, results from several studies in animals and humans have suggested that atherosclerosis, the clogging of blood vessels that can lead to heart attacks or strokes, may be influenced by microbial organisms including viruses such as cytomegalovirus, a herpesvirus family member, and bacteria, such as *Chlamydia, Mycoplasma,* and *Helicobacter pylori.*[9] The latter hypothesis is in line with the change in pathogenetical thinking brought about by the link of a bacterium, *Helicobacter pylori,* to peptic ulcer disease and lymphoma associated with the gastrointestinal mucosa.[75] Therefore, antibiotics have joined antacids in the treatment of some forms of peptic ulcer disease.

The recent molecular biology endeavors that have characterized most of the expressed genes in the human body are opening the doors for using natural proteins with antiviral activity, or even chemical substances directed at the proteins in the body that are the portals of invasion of viruses, as the new weapons in our continuing battle against these microbes. A revisit to old tradition brings to mind some useful paradigms. Many cultures around the world discovered that rubbing a frog on an infected wound would help clear the infection and heal the wound. The small proteins that are responsible for this antibacterial activity in the frog's skin were characterized in the past century. Later, similar proteins were discovered in human beings, some of which also have antiviral activity. Since the genetic makeups and expressed proteins of many different organisms are being deciphered around the world, it is likely that we will continue to discover other natural substances with antiviral activities and maybe even discover those elusive natural enemies of viruses. For instance, one bacterial organism, *Mycoplasma,* has been shown to help the AIDS virus, an observation that supports the hope that there might be another organism that may help kill or control it. In this line of thought, some scientists have proposed that certain populations of people that have proven to be particularly resistant to viral infections despite high-risk behavior may be infected with another organism that confers such protection.

The characterizations of viral genetic makeups, of the proteins that they encode, and of the effects of the latter on cells have also helped to create testing systems for substances present in plants, and it is possible that new chemicals will be derived from the knowledge garnered over centuries in the field of herbal medicine. For instance, Louis Pasteur noted garlic's antibiotic activity in 1858, and, more recently, the sulfur-containing component of garlic, allicin, has been shown to kill all viruses thus far tested in the laboratory.[76] Plant proteins with antiviral activities may also provide templates for the computational biochemistry search for homologous proteins in humans, a task that may help unravel new natural antiviral agents. In fact, over half of the top twenty-five prescription drugs in the market are derived from plants.

Regardless of the source of the drugs, whether naturally occurring or synthetic, the antiviral drug era will continue to open new doors for novel approaches to viral and nonviral diseases. The determination of the sequence of the genome of viruses and of the protein products that they encode has created the targets for a booming pharmaceutical enterprise and represent the first success story of the genomics revolution. Antiviral drugs provide the first glimpse of the exciting new era of molecular medicine, a discipline that welcomes the twenty-first century as an infant for whom we have great expectations. One can only fathom by extrapolation that if the limited number of viral targets so far worked out has generated a number of potential medications that is in the realm of two orders of magnitude the number of targets, at least 1.2 million medications should in the near future be under investigation for the close to 12,000 genes that express secretory proteins in humans. These medications will allow to regenerate failing or aging organs, restore deficient or quell excessive bodily functions, and help combat old and new challenges to human health.

Chapter 2

Viruses As Potential Direct or Indirect Etiological Agents for CFS

As a prelude to the review of antiviral therapies tried for CFS covered in Chapter 3, this chapter summarizes the experience so far garnered in the search for a possible viral etiology of CFS. This chapter also addresses the evidence in favor of a potential autoimmune basis for CFS, possibly as a sequel of a viral infection, as well as the potential role of latent virus reactivation in the etiology and/or perpetuation of CFS.

VIRUSES AS POTENTIAL DIRECT ETIOLOGICAL AGENTS FOR CFS

Several families of viruses have been studied as potential etiological agents of CFS.

Enteroviruses

Enteroviruses (Coxsackie virus A and B, echovirus, poliovirus) belong to a group of small RNA-viruses, picornavirus, which are widespread in nature. Enteroviruses cause a number of well-known diseases and symptoms in humans, from subclinical infections and the common cold to poliomyelitis with paralysis. Serologic and molecular biology techniques have demonstrated that enteroviral genomes, in certain situations, persist after the primary infection, which is often silent. Persistent enteroviral infection or recurrent infections and/or virus-stimulated autoimmunity might contribute to the development of diseases with hitherto unexplained pathogenesis, such as postpolio syndrome, dilated cardiomyopathy, juvenile (type 1) diabetes and possibly some cases diagnosed as CFS.[77-81] Several studies have failed to document persistent enteroviral infections in CFS.[82-84]

Herpesviruses

Herpesviruses (Epstein-Barr virus, cytomegalovirus, human herpes virus types 6 and 7, herpes simplex virus types 1 and 2) have been associated with CFS. For instance, reactivation/replication of a latent herpesvirus (such as Epstein-Barr virus) could modulate the immune system to induce CFS.[85-87] In this respect, serologically proven acute infectious illness secondary to Epstein-Barr virus (EBV) is associated with a range of nonspecific somatic and psychological symptoms, particularly fatigue and malaise rather than anxiety and depression.[88] Although improvement in several symptoms occurs rapidly, fatigue commonly remains a prominent complaint at four weeks, and resolution of fatigue is associated with improvement in cell-mediated immunity. A prospective cohort study of 250 primary care patients also revealed a higher incidence and longer duration of an acute fatigue syndrome and a higher prevalence of CFS after glandular fever as compared to after an ordinary upper respiratory tract infection.[89] In another study, anti-EBV titers were higher among CFS patients and were associated with being more symptomatic.[90] However, testing of 548 chronically fatigued, including patients with CFS, for antibodies to thirteen viruses (herpes simplex virus 1 and 2, rubella, adenovirus, human herpesvirus 6, Epstein-Barr virus, cytomegalovirus, and Coxsackie B virus, types 1 through 6) in patients found no consistent differences in any of the seroprevalences compared with controls.[91]

Some studies suggest an association between human herpesvirus-6 (HHV-6) (*Roseolovirus* genus of the betaherpesvirus subfamily) and CFS.[92-95] One study found that a high proportion of CFS patients (50 percent by antibody testing and up to 80 percent by nested-PCR detection of viral DNA but not RNA) were infected with HHV-6 but with low viral load. The latter results do not support HHV-6 reactivation in CFS patients.[94] Other studies have addressed a possible association between HHV-7 and CFS. Use of the supernatant fluid from HHV-7 infected cells as antigen in immunoassays yielded high and low HHV-7 antibody in sera from chronic fatigue patients and healthy donors as controls, respectively.[96]

Stealth viruses

Cloned DNA obtained from the culture of an African green monkey, simian cytomegalovirus-derived stealth virus contains multiple discrete regions of significant sequence homology to portions of known human cellular genes.[97] The stealth virus has also been cultured from several CFS patients, and a cytopathic stealth virus was also cultured from the cerebrospinal fluid of a nurse with CFS. The findings lend support to the possibility of replicative RNA forms of certain stealth viruses.[98] Review of the clinical histories and brain biopsy findings of three patients with severe stealth virus encephalopathy showed that the patients initially developed symptoms consistent with CFS.[99] One patient has remained in a vegetative state for several years, while the other two patients have shown significant, although incomplete, recovery. Histological and electron-microscopic studies revealed vacuolated cells with distorted nuclei and various cytoplasmic inclusions suggestive of incomplete viral expression. There was no significant inflammatory response. Viral cultures provided further evidence of stealth viral infections occurring in these patients.[99] Partial sequencing of stealth virus segments isolated from a CFS patient revealed a fragmented genome and sequence microheterogeneity, observations that suggest that both the processivity and the fidelity of replication of the viral genome are defective.[100] An unstable viral genome may provide a potential mechanism of recovery from stealth viral illness.

Retroviruses

Some studies[101,102] looked into a possible link between retroviruses and CFS, but no conclusive evidence has been garnered.

Lentiviruses

Although structures consistent in size, shape, and character with various stages of a lentivirus replicative cycle were observed by electron microscopy in twelve-day peripheral-blood lymphocyte cultures from ten of seventeen CFS patients and not in controls, attempts to identify a lymphoid phenotype containing these structures failed and the results of reverse-transcriptase assay of culture supernatant fluids were equivocal.[103]

Parvovirus B19

The spectrum of disease caused by parvovirus B19 has been expanding in recent years because of improved and more sensitive methods of detection. There is evidence to suggest that chronic infection occurs in patients who are not detectably immunosuppressed. A young woman with recurrent fever and a syndrome indistinguishable from CFS was found to have persistent parvovirus B19 viremia, which was detectable by polymerase chain reaction despite the presence of IgM and IgG antibodies to parvovirus B19.[104] Testing of samples from this patient suggested that in some low viremic states, parvovirus B19 DNA is detectable by nested PCR in plasma but not in serum. The patient's fever resolved with the administration of intravenous immunoglobulin.

Ross River Virus

A prospective investigation revealed that serologically proven acute infectious illness due to Ross River virus is associated with a range of nonspecific somatic and psychological symptoms, particularly fatigue and malaise rather than anxiety and depression.[105] Although improvement in several symptoms occurs rapidly, fatigue commonly remains a prominent complaint at four weeks. Resolution of fatigue is associated with improvement in cell-mediated immunity as measured by delayed-type hypersensitivity skin responses.

Borna Disease Virus

Borna disease virus (BDV) is a neurotropic, nonsegmented, negative-sense single-strand RNA virus. Natural infection with this virus has been reported to occur in horses and sheep. Recent epidemiological data suggest that BDV may be closely associated with neuropsychiatric disease (depression and schizophrenia) in humans.[106-113] In Japanese patients with CFS, the prevalence of BDV infection is up to 34 percent. Furthermore, anti-BDV antibodies and BDV RNA were detected in a family cluster with CFS. These results suggest that BDV or a related agent may contribute to or initiate CFS, although the single etiologic role of BDV is unlikely.[106-113]

VIRUSES AS POSSIBLE INDIRECT ETIOLOGICAL AGENTS FOR CFS

Another etiological hypothesis for CFS is that an acute viral infection triggers an autoimmune response; i.e., when the body mounts an attack against the virus, it selects the production of immunoglobulins that can also recognize and attack the body itself. This happens because of what is termed "molecular mimicry." The portions of the virus that the antibodies recognize somehow resemble those of proteins that normally constitute the human body. The evidence for autoimmunity in CFS comes from several sources. One research team found that approximately 52 percent of sera from CFS patients react with nuclear envelope antigens.[114] Some sera from CFS patients immunoprecipitated the nuclear envelope protein lamin B1.[115] Another report documented a high frequency (83 percent) of autoantibodies to insoluble cellular antigens (vimentin and lamin B1) in CFS, a unique feature which might help to distinguish CFS from other rheumatic autoimmune diseases.[116] The possible autoimmune etiology of CFS is further underscored by preliminary evidence for an association between CFS and the presence of HLA-DQ3.[117]

Several studies have documented the presence in CFS patients of rheumatoid factor,[118-125] antinuclear antibodies,[116,118-120,122-127] antithyroid antibodies,[125,128,129] anti–smooth-muscle antibodies,[128] antigliadin, cold agglutinins, cryoglobulins, and false serological positivity for syphilis.[124,128] No circulating antimuscle and anti-CNS antibodies were found in ten CFS patients,[130] and one group found no significant differences in the number of positive tests for autoantibodies in CFS patients.[131]

One team found that among children who chronically complain of nonspecific symptoms such as headache, fatigue, abdominal pain, and low-grade fever, those who were antinuclear antibody (ANA) positive tended to have general fatigue and low-grade fever, while gastrointestinal problems such as abdominal pain and diarrhea and orthostatic dysregulation symptoms were commonly seen in ANA-negative patients.[132] Children who were unable to go to school more than one day a week were seen significantly more among ANA-positive patients than among ANA-negative patients. Based on these observations, the authors concluded that autoimmunity may play a role in childhood chronic nonspecific symptoms and proposed a new disease entity: the autoimmune fatigue syndrome in children.

The features shared between CFS and autoimmune diseases may complicate diagnosis. For instance, three cases of dermatomyositis had been erroneously diagnosed as CFS because of the presence of elevated titers of serum Epstein-Barr virus antibodies.[133] In one study, one-third of CFS patients with sicca symptoms fulfilled the diagnostic criteria for Sjoegren's syndrome, but they were "seronegative," differing from the ordinary primary Sjoegren's syndrome.[134] An additional confounding feature is that patients with primary Sjoegren's syndrome report more fatigue than healthy controls on all the dimensions of the Multidimensional Fatigue Inventory and, when controlling for depression, significant differences remain on the dimensions of general fatigue, physical fatigue, and reduced activity.[135] The negative correlation between levels of noradrenaline and general fatigue in patients with primary Sjoegren's syndrome may imply the involvement of the autonomic nervous system in the chronic fatigue reported in this syndrome.[135,136] Although fatigue in patients with systemic lupus erythematosus (SLE) does not correlate with disease activity, it is correlated with fibromyalgia, depression, and lower overall health status.[137] Fatigue is also a major symptom in patients with ankylosing spondylitis and, unlike SLE, it is more likely to occur with active disease but it may occur as a lone symptom.[138] Fatigue is also common in osteoarthritis and rheumatoid arthritis, associates with measures of distress, and is a predictor of work dysfunction and overall health status.[139] Several studies have reported that rheumatoid arthritis-related fatigue is strongly associated with psychosocial variables, apart from disease activity per se.[140,141] Fatigue is associated to a large extent with pain, self-efficacy toward coping with disease, toward asking for help, and problematic social support, and female gender. One study found large individual differences in variation of pain and fatigue among rheumatoid arthritis patients.[142] Stressors were associated with increased pain but not fatigue. Subjects with poor sleep had higher levels of pain and fatigue. Diurnal cycles of pain and fatigue were found, yet were observed for only some patients.

The increased autoimmune manifestations in CFS, along with the decreased natural killer cell cytotoxic and lymphoproliferative activities, would be compatible with the hypothesis that the immune systems of affected individuals are biased toward a T-helper (Th)2 type, or humoral immunity (antibody producing)-oriented cytokine expression pattern, over a Th1 type, or cellular mediated (natural killer cell and macrophage activating) immunity-oriented one. Potent immunogens can have systemic long-lasting nonspecific effects on the nature of the immune response to unrelated antigens. In particular, vaccinations or infections can exert a systemic effect and nonspecifically increase or reduce the Th1/Th2 cytokine balance of the response to other unrelated antigens[143] and affect (positively or negatively) survival from unrelated diseases.[144,145]

Based on the fact that Gulf War personnel were given multiple Th2-type response-inducing vaccinations, Rook, Stanmford, and Zumla, in international published patent number WO-09826790, present the hypothesis that Gulf War syndrome represents a special case of CFS, where the Th2 inducing stimuli can be identified. The authors point out that induction of a systemic Th2 switch is underscored by four features of the vaccination protocol used for the Gulf War troops:

1. Pertussis was used as an adjuvant in British troops in the Persian Gulf and its adjuvanticity is potently Th2-type response inducing.[146-148] This property of pertussis has recently led to discus-

sion of the possibility that its use in children contributes to the contemporary increased prevalence of atopy.[149,150]

2. Gulf War troops were given Th2-inducing immunogens against plague, anthrax, typhoid, tetanus, and cholera. Such a cumulatively large antigen load would tend to drive the response toward a Th2-type response predominance.[144,151,152] The measles vaccine, when used at the standard dose, reduced mortality by considerably more than can be accounted for by the incidence of measles in the unvaccinated population. It has been reported that diphtheria, tetanus, and pertussis vaccines (Th2 inducing) do not show this nonspecific protective effect.[145] However, when a high titer measles vaccine was used, the mortality increased, although protection from measles itself was maintained.[144,145] There is evidence that this increase in mortality was accompanied by a switch toward a Th2-type response, and dose-related increases in the induction of a Th2 component are well established for several other immunogens.[151,152]

3. The vaccinations were given after deployment of the troops in the war zone or just before they traveled there, at a time when stress levels would have been high. Immunization in the presence of raised levels of glucocorticoids (i.e., cortisol) drives the cytokine expression response by stimulated lymphocytes toward a Th2-type predominance.[153-155] Several steroid hormones modulate T-cell responses. Dehydroepiandrosterone (DHEA) or unknown metabolites of DHEA, tend to promote a Th1-type response pattern. Thus, DHEA can restore immune functions in aged mice through correction of dysregulated cytokine release.[156,157] DHEA has been tested for similar properties in aged humans[158] and found to enhance production of Th1-type cytokines, such as interleukin(IL)-2 and interferon(IFN)-gamma.[159-162] DHEA also enhances IL-2 secretion from human peripheral blood T cells.[163] These effects of DHEA are the reverse of the effects of glucocorticoids, such as cortisol, which enhance Th2-type response activity and synergize with Th2-type cytokines.[164-167] If proliferation of naive T lymphocytes is driven in the presence of a nonspecific stimulus[154] or by an antigen (as follows vaccination), T lymphocytes with a Th2-type cytokine profile will develop. This has been rather clearly shown with spleen cells from laboratory rodents which have few memory cells under normal circumstances.[155] Overall, cortisol favors the

development of a Th2 cytokine profile from naive cells.[154] This point must not be confused with the fact that the cytokine-secreting activity of established Th2-type cells is readily inhibited by cortisol. Thus, the use of cortisol analogs for conventional treatments of Th2-mediated diseases, such as eczema, asthma, and hay fever, may work via anti-inflammatory effects, and by reducing cytokine production by Th2-type cells,[168] and yet at the same time the use of cortisol will encourage perpetuation of the underlying problem by driving newly recruited T cells toward a Th2-type response.

Psychological and physical stress activate the hypothalamic-pituitary-adrenal axis and thereby lead to a variety of changes including increased production of cortisol. In this respect, excessive exercise and deprivation of food and sleep result in a falling ratio of DHEA to cortisol. The latter falling ratio correlates directly with a fall in delayed-type hypersensitivity (DTH) responsiveness (a Th1-type response marker), and there is a simultaneous rise in serum IgE levels. IgE is wholly dependent upon Th2-type cytokine production.[153] This is to be expected in the light of known effects of DHEA and cortisol outlined above. A further example of the effect of stress on Th1- to Th2-type switching is the increase in antibody to Epstein-Barr virus in students reacting in a stressed manner to their exams. This virus is usually controlled by a Th1-type response and cytotoxic T cells. Loss of control results in virus replication and increased antibody production.[169] Similarly, peripheral blood leukocytes from medical students during exam periods showed lower mRNA for IFN-gamma, a Th1-type cytokine.[170] Similar points can be demonstrated in a more controlled manner in animals. Stress secondary to crowding or restraint can increase mycobacterial growth in tuberculous mice.[171,172] This is a model that is acutely sensitive to the presence of even a small Th2 component.[173,174] In tuberculosis, there is a systemic shift to a Th2-type response predominance,[173,174] and an unusual pattern of metabolites of adrenal steroids is excreted in the urine.[174] Treatment of the disease restores the Th1-type predominance and corrects the pattern of steroid metabolites, so that metabolites of cortisone increase relative to metabolites of cortisol.[173,174] There is considerable evidence that depression can be associated with excessive cortisol-mediated effects in the brain,[175,176] and stress can lead to depression. Thus, depression (as seen in CFS and Gulf War syndrome) tends to associate with Th2-mediated disorders, such as asthma, eczema, and some endocrine changes.[177,178] Treatment of depression with the drug metyrapone causes the same change in steroid metabolites (e.g., increase in metabolites of cortisone relative to metabolites of cortisol) as those described above after treatment of tuberculosis.[175,176]

4. The troops were also exposed to carbamate and organophosphorus insecticides, and these inhibit IL-2-driven phenomena essential for normal Th1-type function.[179] The importance of this component is uncertain. However, it has been rumored that the insecticides were often obtained from local sources in the Gulf, so purity was not known, and even more toxic contaminants may have been present.

Thus, multiple vaccinations administered under these circumstances may have caused a long-lasting systemic cytokine imbalance. The same effect would occur sporadically in the general population, secondary to vaccinations or other Th2-type response-inducing environmental stimuli and infections and could account for the widespread incidence of CFS. It should be stressed at this point that not all vaccines and infectious agents induce a preponderance of the Th2-type response. For instance, measles infection reduced the incidence of atopy and of allergic reactions to house dust mite.[143] Similarly, Japanese children that are tuberculin skin-test positive are less likely to be atopic than are tuberculin-negative children, and their ratio of circulating Th1/Th2 cytokines is higher. Moreover, after repeated injection of Bacillus Camelet-Guerin (BCG), those in whom tuberculin conversion occurs have an increased probability of losing their atopic symptoms.

Although vaccines, stressful stimuli, and some pathogens have been shown to lead to long-term nonspecific shifts in cytokine balance,[144-146] the factors that could lead to a Th2 shift in CFS patients are unknown. Nevertheless, as discussed in Chapter 3, several therapeutic regimens which induce a systemic Th1 bias, some based on the use of certain vaccines, are being tested with preliminary success in subpopulations of CFS patients with documented baseline immune abnormalities. Moreover, whether directly or indirectly, viruses may play a role in the etiology or the perpetuation of symptoms of CFS. Some authors have put forth the notion that reactivation of latent viruses, if not etiological, may serve as a perpetuation factor for CFS symptomatology and may account for the remission-exacerbation cycling nature of the disease. On the other hand, viral reactivation may be an epiphenomenon and not necessarily related to symptomatology. Although mainly focused on therapeutic interventions, the following chapter will address the hypotheses discussed above and others on how local and/or systemic effects of acute or reactivated viral activity may underlie CFS.

Chapter 3

Viral-Specific and Immune-Based Nonspecific Antiviral Therapies for CFS

This chapter summarizes the different antiviral therapies thus far tested for CFS, and it addresses their rationale despite lack of clear evidence for a direct or indirect viral etiology of CFS.

ACYCLOVIR AND RELATED ANTIHERPETIC DRUGS

In international published patent number US-058872123, A. M. Lerner reports an approach to alleviate the symptoms of CFS with a therapeutically effective amount of one or more pharmaceutically acceptable antiviral agents selected from the group consisting of acyclovir, ganciclovir, valacyclovir, famciclovir, cidofovir, and pharmaceutically acceptable derivatives and mixtures thereof.

Lerner's premise is that, in general, the clinical symptoms and signs of chronic fatigue syndrome resemble those of infectious mononucleosis. Symptoms common to both illnesses include low-grade fever, chills, sore throat, painful anterior or posterior cervical or axillary lymph nodes, muscle weakness, myalgia, generalized headaches, migratory arthralgia, vague neuropsychological complaints, and disturbances of sleep without known medical cause. As with mononucleosis, a CFS patient's attempt to exercise at levels previously tolerable results in a prolonged and more severe manifestation of the fatigue.

Although CFS and infectious mononucleosis have several similarities, patients with CFS do not have the severe dysphagia and gray exudative pharyngitis often accompanied by submandibular adenopathy, which is associated with infectious mononucleosis and its etiologic agent Epstein-Barr virus (EBV). Lerner's research has found in CFS sufferers the existence of Epstein-Barr virus multiplication, purportedly within epithelial cells of the pharynx and circulating B lymphocytes of the blood. The beta herpes virus, human cytomegalovirus (HCMV), is also believed to cause infectious mononucleosis-type symptoms, without the exudative pharyngitis.

Lerner points out that chronic fatigue syndrome also includes unique symptoms, such as light-headedness or wooziness of varying severity and duration without antecedent cause; a vague, dull, pressure-like chest ache, generally in the substernal region and sometimes including the left shoulder, which is exhibited with increasing fatigue at the end of the day; and palpitations. There is also often a fourth symptom, tachycardia or rapid heart action, even with minimal or no exertion by the sufferer. Based on the symptoms unique to CFS, Lerner further hypothesized that CFS is essentially cardiac in origin, and that this cardiac basis unlocks the key to the disorder.

In the patent publication, Lerner proposes that the majority of CFS cases constitute either a continuing primary herpes virus infection, specifically Epstein-Barr virus and/or human cytomegalovirus or, alternatively, a reactivation infection with latent Epstein-Barr virus and/or latent human cytomegalovirus. In some lesser number of cases, herpes virus 6 (HHV-6) or other viruses, such as enteroviruses, may be involved. Seroepidemiologic studies have documented the presence of EBV and/or HCMV in a significant number of CFS sufferers. Lerner's research has further indicated for CFS sufferers the existence of IgM antibodies to the EBV viral capsid antigen (VCA) or EBV antibodies to early antigen (EA), the latter depicting EBV DNA polymerase activity, which is an indicator of current virus multiplication. In CFS sufferers, there may be additionally or alternatively a significant IgG to HCMV, as detected by enzyme-linked immunosorbent assay (ELISA), with or without an IgM (ELISA) antibody titer to HCMV.

Lerner points out that the understood virologic cause of CFS thus verifies that previous seroepidemiologic studies, attempting to show a singular virologic causation to CFS including singular searches for EBV or HCMV antibodies, would have naturally yielded uniformly negative results. At least fifteen different viruses, bacteria, and parasites have been suspected as singular etiologic agents of CFS. However, there has been, to date, no clear serologic association with any human virus. Lerner proposes that the previous studies were designed in a way that actually masked the possibility of finding a major two-virus causality.

The two major causative herpes viruses proposed by Lerner, EBV and HCMV, are characterized by latent, nonpermissive, persistent infections. In a nonpermissive infection, a complete infectious virus is not produced. Intracellular infection produces a metabolically altered host cell; however, no progeny capable of infecting a new susceptible cell are created. Instead, the extrachromosomal herpes virus episome persists for the life of the chronically infected cell. The latent persistent infection and recrudescent infection characteristic of the herpes virus is common in EBV and HCMV and is consistent with chronic recrudescent illness of CFS.

Productive whole-virus, herpesvirus, EBV, or HCMV infection is accompanied by lysis of infected cells. In latent infection, complete infectious virus is not produced, and host cell survival continues. With persistent infection, varying levels of infectious virus, latent virus, and reactivation may occur simultaneously. Productive infection is also associated with cellular necrosis and a subsequent inflammatory response. Latency may be associated with little inflammation or morphological changes but may lead only to aberrant biochemical and degenerative cellular functions.

Lerner goes on to point out that evidence exists that supports the theory that both HCMV and EBV are cardiotropic for the human myocyte. Based on Lerner's research, the human cardiac myofiber, like the B lymphocyte for EBV and the mononuclear progenitor cell for HCMV, is a site of noninfectious episome-mediated persistent infection. This is different from the human epithelial cell of the pharynx which produces mainly whole infectious EBV virus. HCMV immediate-early gene transcripts have been detected in the heart by in situ hybridization techniques in patients with HIV-associated cardiomyopathy. Likewise, the EBV genome was detected by polymerase chain reaction amplification of DNA extracted from the heart at autopsy. However, polymerase chain reaction for enteroviruses and cardiac viral cultures were negative. An intense mononuclear cell infiltrate in the myocardium consisted essentially of T cells without identifiable B cells.

Accordingly, Lerner's research has suggested that CFS is a nonpermissive, persistent herpesvirus infection of the heart, wherein EBV and/or HCMV nucleic acids are present in the hearts of CFS patients. This hypothesis was generated based in part upon endomyocardial biopsies of patients with CFS. The research conducted revealed that all CFS patients have abnormal oscillating T-wave flattenings and T-wave inversions detectable from twenty-four-hour electrocardiographic (Holter) monitoring. An initial twenty-four-hour electrocardiographic T-wave study compared CFS patients to random non-CFS patients from an internal medicine practice, wherein both patient groups were restricted to an age less than fifty years old to minimize the occurrence of chronic diseases in both populations. Notably, chronic diseases such as hypertensive vascular disease, electrolyte abnormalities, and coronary artery disease may produce similar oscillating abnormal T-waves. However, since people suffering from CFS are generally young, such chronic diseases rarely afflict CFS sufferers and can thus be excluded as the causative agent. Oscillating T-wave abnormalities described also occur in about 5 percent of normal patients when they assume an upright position. For these same patients, in resting twelve-lead standard ECG, T-waves describing left ventricular electrical depolarization are upright, and the resultant ECG is normal. The 2-D echocardiogram also generally is normal, however, the twenty-four-hour ECG recordings (Holter monitoring) are abnormal with oscillating T-wave flattenings or T-wave inversions characteristically incident with the onset of sinus tachycardias and subsequently reverting to normal T-wave configurations with the return of normal sinus rhythms. Although these abnormal T-waves are not specific to CFS, and they occur similarly with diverse conditions such as coronary artery disease, hypertensive vascular disease, and electrolyte abnormalities, the abnormal T-waves detected via Holter monitoring were seen much more frequently in twenty-four random CFS patients than in 116 time-, place-, and age-matched random non-CFS patients. Based on Lerner's analysis, the abnormal T-waves at twenty-four-hour ECG recordings in CFS patients are not artifacts and are a significant sign of CFS. Lerner purports that the abnormal Holter monitoring in CFS patients is evidence that CFS is a cardiomyopathy. Moreover, Lerner has found that the additional symptoms of a dull chest ache coming on at the end of the day not related to exercise, light-headedness or wooziness, and palpitations are CFS symptoms attributable to cardiac involvement by these viruses.

An initial group of CFS patients also demonstrated abnormal left ventricular dynamics characterized by a decreased or falling ejection fraction, abnormal wall motion, or dilatation by radionuclide stress multiple gated acquisition (MUGA) studies. Furthermore, consecutive case series of CFS patients from a single referral center at Birmingham, Michigan, during the years 1987 to 1993 demonstrated abnormal left ventricular dynamic function in 24.1 percent of eighty-seven patients undergoing radionuclide ventriculography by the radioisotopic gated-pool method.

Lerner also reports that, in an effort to diagnose CFS using electron microscopy, cardiomyopathic changes including myofiber hypertrophy, myofiber disarray, and degenerative change in myofibers have been seen. On rare occasions, inflammatory myocarditis is evident. Infectious HCMV is not found in the heart, peripheral blood, or urine of the HCMV-infected CFS subset of patients. Based on evidence gathered, Lerner conclusively believes that CFS is a major newly discovered cardiomyopathy. Lerner has also observed that patients with acute primary EBV infectious mononucleosis who recover rapidly have normal Holter monitoring throughout their illnesses. Lerner also argues that just like CFS, herpes simplex virus encephalitis boggled the medical community because etiologic identification due to the rising antibodies in serum may or may not be present at a particular time. Diagnosis of this form of encephalitis required isolation of herpes simplex virus type 1 (HSV-1) from the brains of patients with encephalitis.

Because the herpes viruses are intracellular parasites which use multiple biochemical pathways of the infected host cell, initially there were problems associated with achieving clinically useful antiviral activity without also adversely affecting normal host cell metabolism and causing toxicity. Therefore, as pointed out in Chapter 1, acyclovir, as a selective inhibitor of herpes simplex virus multiplication, represented an important advance in antiviral therapy. Acyclovir was synthesized in 1974 by Beauchamp and Schaeffer of Burroughs-Wellcome Company. Acyclovir, 9-([2-hydroxyethoxy]methyl) guanine E, demonstrated significant in vitro antiviral activity against herpesviruses, specifically, HSV, varicella zoster virus (VZV), and EBV.

Acyclovir is an acyclic analog of guanosine. The inhibitory activity of acyclovir is highly selective. The enzyme thymidine kinase (TK) of normal uninfected cells does not effectively use acyclovir as a substrate. However, TK encoded by the herpes simplex virus converts acyclovir into acyclovir monophosphate, a nucleotide analog. The monophosphate is further converted into diphosphate by cellular guanylate kinase and into triphosphate by a number of cellular enzymes. Acyclovir triphosphate interferes with herpes simplex virus DNA polymerase and inhibits viral replication. Acyclovir is preferentially taken up and selectively converted to the active triphosphate form by herpes virus-infected cells. Acyclovir triphosphate binds viral DNA polymerase, acting as a DNA chain terminator. Because acyclovir is taken up selectively by virus-infected cells, the concentration of acyclovir triphosphate is forty to 100 times higher in infected cells than in uninfected cells. Furthermore, viral DNA polymerase exhibits a ten- to thirtyfold greater affinity for acyclovir triphosphate than do cellular DNA polymerases. The higher concentration of the active triphosphate metabolite in infected cells plus the affinity for viral polymerases result in the very low toxicity of acyclovir for normal host cells.

Although EBV and HCMV do not have virus-specific TKs, replication of the EBV and HCMV DNA is significantly impaired. Acyclovir's in vitro antiviral activity is considerably greater in HSV than HCMV. More recently, Burroughs Wellcome has introduced Valtrex (valacyclovir hydrochloride) the hydrochloride salt of the L-valyl ester of acyclovir. Valacyclovir is preferred because of its high bioavailability. As a result of valacyclovir's increased absorption, as compared to acyclovir, for example, less frequent dosages of valacyclovir are required to reach effective antiherpetic levels. Another antiviral agent, ganciclovir, or 9-(1,3-dihydroxy-2-propoxymethyl)guanine, has increased in vitro activity against all herpes viruses as compared to acyclovir, including an eight to twenty times greater activity against HCMV. However, toxicity concerns prevent the use of gancyclovir for a relatively benign HCMV infection.

Another effective antiviral agent is Vistide, or cidofovir, 1-[(s)-3-hydroxy-2-(phosphomethoxy) propyl]cytosine dihydrate. Cidofovir also suppresses replication of the herpes viruses by selective inhibition of viral DNA synthesis. Cidofovir is incorporated into the growing viral DNA chain, a process which results in reductions in the rate of viral DNA synthesis.

Famvir, famciclovir, the 6-deoxy analog of the active antiviral compound penciclovir, is also believed to have antiviral activity against HSV-1 and VZV. Several additional compounds have demonstrated activity against the herpes viruses. For instance, foscarnet sodium (trisodium phosphonoformate) a pyrophosphate analog of phosphonoacetic acid, has potent in vitro and in vivo activity against herpes viruses. Foscarnet inhibits the DNA polymerase of all human herpes viruses by blocking the pyrophosphate binding site which prevents chain elongation. Bromovinyl arabinosyl uracil has also exhibited significant inhibition of HSV-1, EBV, and VZV. Fluoroiodoarabinosyl cytosine and its related compounds offer another potent inhibitor of herpes viruses. Like acyclovir, the activity of the latter antiviral agent depends on phosphorylation by herpes virus TK. However, this antiviral agent and its analogs appear to have greater activity than acyclovir and significant activity against VZV and HCMV. (S)-1-((3-hydroxy-2-phosphonyl methoxy) propyl)adenine (HPMPA) is yet another antiviral agent which includes a new class of nucleotide analogs with in vitro activity against HSV-1 and -2, HCMV, VZV, and EBV.

Lerner recommends valacyclovir and ganciclovir as the preferred antiviral agents for CFS treatment because the etiologic agents are proposed to be EBV or HCMV. In his studies in the published patent, ten CFS patients, in whom singular EBV persistent infection was demonstrated, were treated with an oral dose of valacyclovir at 10 mg/kg every six hours and studied over a three-month period. EBV active infection was demonstrated by EBV

VCA IgM antibodies and/or elevated EBV EA antibody titers. Each patient's functional status was recorded as a statistically validated energy index (EI). A patient with a 0 EI is bedridden; with an energy index of 1 or 2, any activity by the patient leads to overwhelming, incapacitating fatigue; patients with an energy index between 3 and 5 can, with great effort, be out of bed for several hours each day doing nonphysical activities; patients with an energy index between 6 and 9 can assume normal activities and maintain a forty-hour workweek and, with pacing, maintain a household; and patients with an energy index of 10 have normal energy levels, stamina, and a sense of well-being. The mean baseline EI for the ten CFS patients with EBV was 4.6, and the EI range was 3.5 to 5.5. At the completion of therapy, the same CFS patients had a mean EI of 7.5, a median EI of 7, and a range between 6 and 10. Prior to therapy, five of the ten patients had chest pain. At the completion of the trial, one of the ten patients had chest pain. At the beginning of the trial, nine of the ten patients had lightheadedness, unsteadiness, and inability to think well. At the completion of the trial, one of the ten patients continued to have these symptoms. At the beginning of the trial, five of the ten patients had palpitations, while at the completion of the trial, three of the ten patients had palpitations. At the completion of the trial, eight of the ten patients continued to have positive EA antibody titers.

Another study was conducted to assess the possible efficacy of ganciclovir treatment on a subset of CFS patients with high HCMV IgG ELISA antibody titers; minimal/no serologic evidence of concurrent EBV multiplication; and oscillating ECG abnormalities at Holter monitoring. From March 1993 through June 1994, three men and fifteen women with mean age of 39.7 ± 7.7 years, with CFS, were recruited from a single infectious diseases referral center in Birmingham, Michigan. The eighteen CFS patients had a duration of overwhelming fatigue of more than two years and with oscillating or repetitively abnormal aberrant T-waves at twenty-four-hour ECG recordings using Holter monitoring. In these eighteen CFS patients, baseline standard 12 lead ECG, 2-D echocardiogram, rest-stress myocardial perfusion (thallium 201 or Tc-99 cardiolite) and rest-stress multiple gated acquisitions (MUGA) studies as well as coronary angiography excluded coronary artery disease. After placement of a peripheral inserted central catheter or a Groshong catheter, ganciclovir was given intravenously in a dose of 5 mg/kg at twelve-hour intervals for thirty days. After thirty days, patients were seen at intervals of four to six weeks and evaluated at each of these times. Of the eighteen patients, thirteen improved and resumed their normal pre-CFS activity levels. The mean duration of fatigue prior to therapy was longer in the five patients who did not improve (2.8 years) than in the fifteen who did improve (mean of 1.6). Prior to receiving intravenous ganciclovir, patients who improved as well as those who did not experienced marked worsening fatigue with exercise, myalgia, light-headedness, and dull, nonspecific, left-sided chest aches not related to activity. After treatment with ganciclovir, three of the fifteen patients who improved with previously abnormal myocardial dynamics reverted to normal, and in three others, results of MUGA tests improved with lesser degrees of tardokinesis, hypokinesis, or left ventricular dilatation. Right ventricular endomyocardial biopsies showing varying degrees of cardiomyopathic changes characterized by myofiber disarray, myofiber dissolution, myofiber drop out with fibrous replacement, and occasioned myofiber hypertrophy were evident in seven of the fourteen patients. There were no adverse events or symptoms attributable to ganciclovir. In an initial test, a single patient had a transient increase in serum creatinine, but upon recalculation of dosage based upon lean body mass in a repeated test, the serum creatinine level reverted to normal.

Lerner also presented a case report in his patent filing. A fifty-one-year-old millwright, who enjoyed excellent health and whose only risk factor for coronary artery disease was cigarette smoking, suddenly experienced overwhelming, progressive fatigue forcing him to stop work. As a result of this fatigue, he was essentially bedridden and slight exertion further worsened his fatigue. He suffered from light-headedness, generalized muscle aches, intermittent sore throat, and an inability to think clearly. The physical exam was normal, chest X ray, HDL cholesterol levels, and urinalysis were normal. A resting 12-lead ECG showed an inverted T-wave in standard lead III, but was otherwise normal. An IgM antibody titer to HCMV was positive, while Epstein-Barr virus antibody tests were negative. Holter monitoring showed oscillating abnormal flat or inverted T-waves appearing with the onset of sinus tachycardias, and alternating with the reappearance of normal upright T-waves when tachycardias resolved. A myocardial sestamibi perfusion rest/stress test showed reversible ischemia of the anterior, apical, and inferior walls, but at cardiac catheterization, the coronary arteries were patent. A stress MUGA study revealed abnormal left ventricular function with a resting ejection fraction of 40 percent (normal >50 percent).

This patient was given daily intravenous ganciclovir treatment at 5 mg/kg every twelve hours for thirty days. Five months later, the stress MUGA test was repeated and, at this time, the resting ejection fraction had increased 14 percent, from 40 to 54 percent, a normal level. Five months later, the patient's maximal cardiac ejection fraction increased from 54 to 68 percent. At this time, repeat myocardial perfusion studies during exercise were normal. Left ventricular dysfunction was no longer present, and the patient's fatigue had disappeared. Subsequently, the patient resumed work as a millwright and, after a 2.5 year follow-up, remains well with normal left ventricular function.

Based on the results described above, Lerner concludes that CFS patients with a significant IgG HCMV antibody titer greater than 120 units, with or without the presence of an IgM HCMV ELISA antibody titer plus an absence of EBV VCA IgM antibody titer, along with an EBV EA antibody titer less than 40, describes a group of CFS patients that should benefit from ganciclovir treatment.

AMPLIGEN

Ampligen, a form of mismatched double-stranded RNA (dsRNA) with immunostimulatory and antiviral activity, is under development by HEMISPHERx BIOPHARMA, INC., primarily for the potential treatment of chronic fatigue syndrome or myalgic encephalomyelitis. It is in Phase III trials in the United States for this indication. HEMISPHERx and its licensing partner, Bioclone, initiated this year the use of Ampligen for severe CFS on a named patient, cost recovery basis in South Africa. It is also under study for other viral infections including hepatitis-B virus (HBV), hepatitis-C virus (HCV), and HIV.

Based on the premise that the clinical symptoms of CFS could be explained by a persistent viral infection, some researchers have reasoned that alterations in the 2',5'-oligoadenylate (2-5) synthetase/RNase L antiviral pathways may underlie CFS.[180,181] This double-stranded RNA (dsRNA)-dependent, interferon-inducible pathway is part of the antiviral defense mechanism of mammalian cells which also regulates cell growth and differentiation.[182-185] When activated by dsRNA, 2-5A synthetase converts ATP to 2',5'-linked oligoadenylates. These biologically active 2-5A molecules bind to and activate a latent endoribonuclease (RNase L) to hydrolyze single-stranded viral and cellular RNA, thus inhibiting protein synthesis.

Various studies have demonstrated that several key components of the 2-5A synthetase/RNase L pathway are significantly dysregulated in CFS.[186-188] In CFS, 2-5A synthetase is predominantly in its activated form.[186,187] In addition, bioactive 2-5A levels are significantly elevated and RNase L activity is upregulated compared to healthy controls.[186,187] A report has also documented 80, 42, and 37 kDa 2-5A binding proteins that possess 2-5A-dependent RNase L enzyme activity in extracts of peripheral blood mononuclear cells from individuals with CFS.[188] These 2-5A binding proteins have been identified by photoaffinity labeling with an azido 2-5A photoprobe, immunoprecipitation with a highly purified, recombinant, human 80 kDa RNase L-specific polyclonal antibody and Phosphor-Imager analysis of SDS-PAGE under denaturing conditions. The 80 kDa RNase L and the 37 kDa low molecular weight (LMW) RNase L proteins bind 2-5A and have 2-5A-dependent RNase L enzyme activity following fractionation by analytical gel permeation high-performance liquid chromatography (HPLC) under native (nondenaturing) conditions.[188]

Suhadolnik and colleagues[180] reported that both RNase L activity and bioactive 2-5A concentration are negatively correlated with Karnofsky performance score in CFS patients. RNase L activity also positively correlated with a second clinical measure, the Metabolic Screening Questionnaire (MSQ), an observation that suggests that the upregulation of the 2-5A synthetase/RNase L pathways is an indication of a lower state of general health. A strong correlation between IFN-alpha and LMW RNase L in a subset of the highest 100 IFN-alpha values from all study subjects is consistent with a viral etiology of CFS.[180]

A highly significant correlation between the 80 kDa RNase L and the LMW RNase levels in CFS patients suggests that the LMW RNase L may be derived form the 80 kDa RNase L. Several lines of biochemical evidence are consistent with the possibility that a cellular or virus-encoded protease may be involved in the origin of the LMW RNase L.[180] Numerous proteases have been demonstrated to have a functional impact in normal and virus-infected cells. One such example is PKR which is hydrolyzed by a protease encoded by the poliovirus genome.[181] A second example is exemplified in the report that proteins in muscle extracts (i.e., actin and myosin) are found to be degraded via ubiquitin-dependent pathways.[189] This degradative process provides amino acids for hepatic gluconeogenesis. For proteins implicated in the control of cell growth and differentiation, such as RNase L, proteolytic degradation in a ubiquitin-dependent manner would protect the cell from formation of abnormal proteins. A third example is proteolytic degradation occurring via the proinflammatory cytokines, IFN-alpha and tumor necrosis factor (TNF)-alpha. TNF-alpha levels have been reported to be elevated in individuals with CFS compared to controls.[190-193] IFN-alpha and TNF-alpha together induce the activity of 2-5A synthetase which ultimately results in the selective degradation of 28S ribosomal RNA, a substrate for RNase L.[194] TNF-alpha may facilitate formation of the LMW RNase L from the 80 kDa RNase L to augment the inhibition of protein synthesis by hydrolyzing RNA.

Through the mechanisms described above, the mismatched double-stranded RNA in Ampligen stimulates production of tumor necrosis factor, interferons, and other lymphokines and has anticancer effects, as does matched double-stranded RNA, but the mismatched version does not share many of the toxic effects of the matched version. Ampligen crosses the blood-brain barrier and shows no rebound effects after withdrawal and has greater antiviral activity than the interferons, one of the cell's natural antiviral signaling systems. Nevertheless, an initial application to the FDA by HEM Pharmaceuticals, the predecessor to HEMISPHERx, for expanded distribution of Ampligen for treatment of CFS was suspended due to cited life-threatening side effects, including hepatic toxicity, severe abdominal pain, and irregular heartbeat.

In 1998, HEMISPHERx received authorization from the U.S. Food and Drug Administration to commence a confirmatory placebo-controlled, multicentered, Phase III study of Ampligen in CFS patients. This confirmatory study commenced in August 1998, with patients enrolled at an investigational site in San Diego. The protocol was for a twenty-four-week period in a placebo-controlled, double-blinded trial involving 230 patients. Contractual agreements with further sites in October 1998, January 1999, and May 1999 brought the total number of sites participating in the Phase III trial to eight.

After an encouraging open-label trial, a placebo-controlled, double-blind, multicenter trial, involving ninety-two subjects, was conducted. After twenty-four weeks of Ampligen treatment, there were significant improvements in physical performance as measured by the primary endpoint, the Karnofsky performance score (KPS), which increased by 43 percent from 53 to 76. Secondary endpoints, which were also met, included reduced cognitive deficit (as assessed by the cognitive subscale of SCL 90-R or neuropsychological function tests); enhanced capacity to perform activities of everyday living; and improvements on treadmill testing (oxygen uptake increased from 1.16 L/min to 1.48 L/min). Notably, a significant reduction in the need for other medications and for extended hospital stays were also observed.

HEMISPHERx reviewed physical performance, cognition, and quality of life improvements derived from Ampligen treatment in four separate clinical studies at the October 10, 1998, session of the American Association for Chronic Fatigue Syndrome Research Conference. The clinical trials reviewed in the presentation include three open-label studies and one placebo-controlled study. These studies indicated that Ampligen has a favorable safety profile and is well tolerated in primates. In addition, long-term Ampligen patients did not reveal any cardiac abnormalities attributable to the drug; adverse effects occurred in 15 percent of patients most of which involved occasional skin flushing and dry skin. Beyond this, the number of adverse effects reported by Ampligen patients was not significantly different from those receiving placebo.

In September 1999, HEMISPHERx announced the results of a pharmacoeconomic study which showed considerable cost-benefits of using Ampligen, in particular, a reduction in the doses used of other medicines and in the number of days spent in the hospital. Results from a separate study showed that the duration of Ampligen positive results remained constant for forty-two months after the start of therapy.

A full new drug application (NDA) to the European Medical Evaluation Agency (EMEA) was submitted in December 1998, with enrollment for a confirmatory Phase II European trial for CFS to support U.S. data and was expected to begin the first quarter of 1999. In February 1999, the company's European marketing application for the treatment of CFS cleared the first stage of regulatory review by being designated as complete by the EMEA. The European Union marketing application was withdrawn in April 2000 following HEMISPHERx's signing of a more economically viable manufacturing agreement for the drug. The company expects to file again.

2CVV

In October 1995, Milkhaus Laboratory, Inc., initiated a Phase I/II clinical trial of 2CVV for the treatment of chronic fatigue syndrome at the Rhode Island Hospital and the Roger Williams Hospital (Brown University affiliates). The trial was completed and 2CVV is available to patients under a compassionate use program. The compound is also in preclinical evaluation for potential treatment of herpes and cystic fibrosis. No published scientific information is available on this compound and Milkhaus is seeking codevelopment partners worldwide.

EPSTEIN-BARR VIRUS VACCINE

Aviron and GlaxoSmithKline reported their collaboration on the development of an Epstein-Barr virus vaccine using Aviron's subunit vaccine technology and GlaxoSmithKline's adjuvant technology. The vaccine was expected to have potential in chronic fatigue syndrome and infectious mononucleosis. A Phase I trial, with two intramuscular injectable formulations, commenced in December 1997 in Belgium. The randomized, double-blind trial in sixty-seven subjects showed the vaccine to be safe and well tolerated. Laboratory tests showed evidence of immune response in the vaccine recipients. No further reports on this vaccine are available.

IMUNOVIR (INOSINE PRANOBEX)

A pilot study of the clinical impact of the synthetic purine derivative imunovir in sixteen CFS patients revealed enhanced natural killer cell activity and clinical improvement in 60 percent of the patients studied. Ardern Healthcare's Imunovir has immunomodulating and antiviral properties and is currently registered for the treatment of acute and chronic viral infections including herpes and measles. Although the product had also been in development for preventing and delaying progression of AIDS in patients at the early stages of the disease, the efficacy for this indication was questioned and the application for European Union approval was withdrawn in 1991. Besides CFS, Imunovir is being studied for the treatment of hepatitis C and infections caused by human papillomavirus.

INFLUENZA VIRUS VACCINE ALONE
OR IN COMBINATION WITH OTHER VACCINES

The use of the influenza virus vaccine and the rubella virus vaccine both separately and together have been reported for the treatment of herpes virus (Epstein-Barr virus) infections. Lieberman[195] reported the use of influenza virus vaccine given together with histamine and the immune enhancer Staphage Lysate for the treatment of patients suffering from Epstein-Barr virus infection. Patients were also successfully treated with the latter mixture in combination with rubella virus vaccine and with rubella virus vaccine alone.

McMichael reported relief of lesion pain and lesion enlargement upon treatment of patients with recurrent herpes simplex virus type II infection with compositions including histamine, measles inactivated, attenuated virus, and influenza vaccine (killed) virus. In published patent number U.S. 4,880,626, McMichael presents a composition for alleviating the symptoms of AIDS comprising human chorionic gonadotropin, Staphage Lysate, an influenza virus vaccine, such as Fluogen, and fractionated inactivated HIV virus. McMichael later reported that the thimerosal preservative in influenza vaccine preparations can mediate the antiherpetic activity of the latter composition (see under thimerosal).

INTERFERON-ALPHA

As mentioned above, interferons are soluble immune mediators involved in natural antiviral defenses. Amarillo Biosciences, Inc. (Amarillo, Texas), conducted a Phase II clinical study with interferon (IFN)-alpha in fibromyalgia patients. The study was designed to measure the effectiveness of low doses of orally administered IFN-alpha in relieving morning stiffness of joints, a significant problem for fibromyalgia sufferers. Although improvement was more pronounced in patients taking one lozenge containing 50 international units of IFN-alpha once daily, the result did not reach statistical significance relative to controls. Increasing the dosage to three IFN-alpha lozenges per day did not improve the results. A confounder for the analysis and interpretation of the results from the latter study is the fact that all participants were given a low dose of the antidepressant drug amitriptyline, which they began taking one month before the start of the IFN-alpha trial and continued throughout the three-month study.

Several companies developed various forms of IFNs, that have been approved and are available in regional markets, with features that may help to overcome the limitations of the study described above. BioNative AB is marketing IFN-alpha subtypes as IFN Alfanative in Sweden, and Mochida Pharmaceutical Co., Ltd., and LG Chemical, Ltd., are marketing their IFN-alpha and IFN-beta in the Far East. Hoffmann-La Roche, Inc., is developing chemically modified forms of IFN-alpha by coupling large polyethylene glycol molecules (PEG) to its IFN-alfa2alpha. Roche calls this conjugate Pegasys and it appears to have improved pharmacokinetic and pharmadynamic activities compared to the company's currently available IFN-alfa2alpha (Roferon-A). Thus, Pegasys is expected to significantly improve efficacy while providing the convenience of once-a-week treatment. Pegasys is currently in Phase III clinical trials for the treatment of chronic hepatitis C and it is also expected to be effective in the treatment of certain cancers. Pepgen Corp. is also developing several mutant forms of human IFN-alpha that have potent antiviral activities but are less toxic than currently available forms of IFN-alpha. Pepgen Corp. expects to file an investigational new drug (IND) for a mutant form of IFN-alpha in 2000.

Pepgen Corp. is also developing an ovine form of IFN called IFN-tau. There is no human homolog to IFN-tau; however, this cytokine was found to have potent antiviral activity and antiproliferative activity against a wide range of human cell lines at concentrations similar to those of IFN-alpha. Structurally, IFN-tau is about 45 to 55 percent homologous with IFN-alpha from human, mouse, rat, or pig. IFN-tau has two potential advantages over currently available IFNs that have been demonstrated in animal studies: first, it was found to be orally available, and, second, it was significantly less toxic than either IFN-alpha or IFN-beta. IFN-tau is in Phase I clinical trials.

JUZEN-TAIHO-TO

A group of Japanese herbal medicines called Hozai have been used to improve the physical condition of the elderly. One representative Hozai, Juzen-Taiho-To, was shown to modulate antigen-specific T-cell responses toward more balanced Th1/Th2-type responses in old BALB/c mice, which have a preferential Th2-type cytokine response pattern.[196] Such effects may help prevent the development of diseases associated with immunodysregulation, including chronic fatigue syndrome.

LYMPH NODE CELL-BASED IMMUNOTHERAPY

Nancy Klimas, Mary Ann Fletcher, and Roberto Patarca at the University of Miami, completed a safety and feasibility study using lymph node extraction, ex vivo cell culture, followed by autologous cell reinfusion as a treatment strategy to favor a Th2- to Th1-type cytokine expression shift in selected CFS patients.[197] Lymph nodes were obtained from patients who met the current case definition for CFS and the following inclusion criteria: a history of acute onset; a Karnofsky performance score less than 80; evidence of immune dysfunction in three or more of the following: greater than one standard deviation above controls for elevated soluble TNF receptor type I (sTNF-RI) levels in serum, elevated sTNF-RI production in phytohemagglutinin (PHA)-stimulated blood culture, or elevated IL-5 production in PHA-stimulated blood culture; lymphocyte activation (CD2 + CD26 + cells > 50 percent); or low NK cell cytotoxic activity (<20 percent). The lymph node cells were cultured for ten to twelve days with anti-CD3 and IL-2. These cells were then reinfused into the donor who was monitored for safety and possible clinical benefit. There were no adverse events noted in this Phase I clinical trial. Of thirteen subjects, two had palpable lymph nodes that proved fibrotic with no viable cells. Of the remaining eleven subjects, all successfully underwent expansion and reinfusion. In some of the patients, there was an elevation in the expression of IL-2 receptor on CD4 T cells in the weeks following the reinfusion. There was a significant decrease in IL-5 production by PHA-stimulated blood cultures observed at one week which persisted for several weeks postinfusion. Levels of PHA-induced IFN-gamma did not change. There was a trend toward a decrease in the ratio of IFN-gamma/IL-5 starting at week one and persisting at least twelve weeks postinfusion. Of the eleven subjects in the trial who had cells reinfused, nine had significant cognitive improvement; other measures of severity of illness also trended toward improvement. The lack of adverse effects from this experimental approach to immunomodulation in CFS and the favorable clinical and immunologic results observed in the small number of patients studied suggest that further clinical trials are warranted.

These studies on CFS patients were preceded by studies of adoptive CD8+ T-cell immunotherapy of AIDS patients with Kaposi's sarcoma.[198-203] The research group used a device developed to selectively capture CD8+ T cells for ex vivo culture and instituted basic science and clinical evaluations of the consequences of the infusion, with rIL-2, of autologous, activated, and polyclonally expanded CD8+ T cells in AIDS patients with Kaposi's sarcoma and oral hairy leukoplakia. Phase I and II trials showed safety and suggested efficacy in the treatment of the latter AIDS associated conditions. The intervention affected the patterns of cytokine expression of CD8+ T lymphocytes and favored a restoration of a strong type 1 response.[203]

MYCOBACTERIUM VACCAE

As described in international published patent number WO-09826790 by Rook, Stanford, and Zumla, preparations of killed *Mycobacterium vaccae* are able to effect a nonspecific systemic Th1-type response bias, in particular by downregulation of Th2-type activity without concomitant upregulation of Th1-type activity. The latter feature is similar to the effect on the Th1/Th2 proportions of the lymph node cell-based immunotherapy previously described.

In experimental animals, a nonspecific systemic bias away from Th2-type activity on administration of *M. vaccae* can be seen as a reduction in the titer of an IL-4 (Th2)-dependent antibody response to ovalbumin (an allergen unrelated to *M. vaccae* itself), in mice preimmunized so as to establish a Th2-type response. A single injection of *M. vaccae* is able to cause this effect, and further injections can enhance it. The effect is nonspecific because it does not require the presence of any component of ovalbumin in the injected preparation.

Briefly, BALB/c mice six to eight weeks old were immunized with 50 μg ovalbumin emulsified in oil (incomplete Freund's adjuvant) on days 0 and 24. This is known to evoke a strong Th2-type pattern of response, accompanied by IgE production, and priming for release of two Th2-type cytokines, IL-4 and IL-5. Animals then received saline or 10^7 autoclaved *M. vaccae* on days 53 and 81 by subcutaneous injection. Injections of *M. vaccae* reduced the rise in IgE levels caused by immunization with ovalbumin. The reduction caused by treatment with *M. vaccae* was significant at all time points tested. Similarly, spleen cells from the immunized animals failed to release IL-5 in vitro in response to ovalbumin if the donor animals had been treated with *M. vaccae,* while spleen cells from immunized animals treated with saline released large quantities of IL-5 in response to ovalbumin. The latter data show that *M. vaccae* will reduce a Th2-type pattern of response, even when given after immunization with a potent allergen and without epitopes of the Th2-inducing molecule. There is therefore a nonspecific systemic downregulation of the Th2-type pattern of response, not dependent upon a direct adjuvant effect on the allergen itself.

In cancer patients, the effect of *M. vaccae* injection has been demonstrated by the appearance in the peripheral blood of lymphocytes that spontaneously secrete IL-2 (a characteristic Th1 cytokine) and decrease in T cells that secrete IL-4 (a characteristic Th2 cytokine) after stimulation with phorbol myristate acetate and calcium ionophore. The percentage of lymphocytes showing this activated Th1-type phenotype increases progressively after each successive injection of *M. vaccae,* reaching a plateau in many individuals after three to five injections of 10^9 organisms (days 0, 15, 30, and then monthly).

The *M. vaccae* used for these therapies is grown on a solid medium including modified Sauton's medium solidified with 1.3 percent agar. The medium is inoculated with the microorganisms and incubated aerobically for ten days at 32°C to enable growth of the microorganism to take place. The microorganisms are then harvested and weighed and suspended in diluent to give 100 mg of microorganisms/mL of diluent. The suspension is then further diluted with buffered saline to give a suspension containing 10 mg wet weight (about 10^{10} cells) of microorganisms/mL of diluent and dispensed into 5 mL multidose vials. The vials containing the live microorganisms are then autoclaved (115 to 125°C) for ten minutes at 69 kPa to kill the microorganisms. The therapeutic agent thus produced is stored at 4°C before use. Then 0.1 mL of the suspension, containing 1 mg wet weight (about 10^9 cells) of

M. vaccae, is shaken vigorously immediately before being administered by intradermal injection over the left deltoid muscle.

In the same patent publication, Rook, Stamford, and Zumla describe their experience with CFS patients treated with *M. vaccae.* For instance, a CFS patient reported improvement after two injections of a *M. vaccae* preparation. A second one reported that since she had been receiving a *M.vaccae* preparation at two-month intervals, her CFS symptoms and food allergy had improved considerably and she feels very well as long as she continues with her regular injections.

PANAX GINSENG

In one study, an extract of the herb *Panax ginseng* was evaluated for its capacity to stimulate cellular immune function by peripheral blood mononuclear cells (PBMC) from normal individuals and patients with chronic fatigue syndrome. PBMC isolated on a Ficoll-Hypaque density gradient were tested in the presence or absence of varying concentrations of the extract for natural killer (NK) cell cytotoxic activity directed against K562 cell targets and for antibody-dependent cellular cytotoxicity (ADCC) directed against human herpesvirus 6-infected H9 cells.[204] Ginseng, at concentrations greater or equal to 10 µg/kg, significantly enhanced NK cell function in both groups. Similarly, the addition of the herb significantly increased ADCC of PBMC from the subject groups. Thus, an extract of *Panax ginseng* enhances cellular immune function of PBMC from normal individuals as well as from patients with depressed cellular immunity and chronic fatigue syndrome.[204] In line with the latter observations, ginseng treatment was found in another study to lead to activation of neutrophils and modulation of the immunoglobulin G response to *Pseudomonas aeruginosa,* thereby enhancing the bacterial clearance and reducing the formation of immune complexes, effects which resulted in a milder lung pathology in chronic *Pseudomonas aeruginosa* lung infection in cystic fibrosis patients. The therapeutic effects of ginseng may be related to activation of a Th1-type of cellular immunity and downregulation of humoral immunity.[205]

Although ginseng is generally well tolerated, it has been implicated as a cause of decreased response to warfarin and may interfere with either digoxin pharmacodynamically or with digoxin monitoring.[206-208] Nevertheless, some authors claim no relationship between cardiac glycosides and glycosides in ginseng and attribute the effect on digoxin on contaminants.[209,210] In addition, ginseng may cause headache, tremulousness, and manic episodes in patients treated with phenelzine sulfate. Ginseng should also not be used with estrogens or corticosteroids because of possible additive effects. Ginseng may affect blood glucose levels and should not be used in patients with diabetes mellitus.[207]

SIZOFIRAN

Sizofiran, an immunostimulant extracted from suehirotake mushroom *(Schizophyllum commune)* cultured fluid, is under development by Fidia Farmaceutici Italiani Deriviate Industriali e Affini for the potential treatment of cancer and hepatitis B. Sizofiran is licensed by Kaken Pharmaceutical Co., Ltd., Japan. Trials were underway for the treatment of gastric and lung tumor; Phase III trials are underway for the treatment of hepatitis B; and the compound is in Phase II trials for chronic fatigue syndrome. By August 1999, Kaken was preparing its NDA filing for hepatitis B.

Significant sizofiran-induced rises in IFN-gamma and IL-2 in culture medium of phytohemagglutinin (PHA) or concanavalin A-stimulated peripheral blood mononuclear cells have been observed. Further reports on sizofiran should become available in the near future.

SPV-30

Arkopharma SA (France) carried out clinical trials on the tree (boxwood) extract, SPV-30, as a natural health product with potential for the treatment of AIDS or chronic fatigue syndrome. SPV-30 is a reverse transcriptase inhibitor and TNF-alpha antagonist. Although SPV-30 use was reported to be safe and to be associated with improvements in CD4 and CD8 cells, energy levels, appetite, memory, weight, and viral load, and a Phase III clinical trial of SPV-30 was completed in 1996, the company has not carried out further trials since that time and plans no further development.

STAPHYLOCOCCAL VACCINE

In international published patent number WO-09829133 by Goteborg University Science Invest AB, Carl-Gerhard Gottfries and Bjorn Regland describe the use of staphylococcal vaccine to favor a Th-1-type predominance. The treatment is preferably conducted as a series of administrations with increasing doses during a specific period. Preferably, the vaccine is administered in eight to ten increasing doses during four to twelve weeks, preferably eight to ten weeks. The reason for the increasing doses is that during the first week or weeks, the patient will probably suffer from side effects, and it is therefore advantageous to start with a low dose. The side effects will diminish after some time. The first series of administrations is followed by repeated administrations given approximately once a week for five to fifteen weeks, preferably for ten weeks. To prevent recurrence, the repeated administrations are then followed by a maintenance treatment with administrations approximately once a month, which preferably are continued for several years, such as one to ten years, preferably approximately five years. The doses in the repeated administrations of the maintenance treatment are preferably constant and relatively high. Vitamin B_{12} and/or folacin is preferably administered simultaneously or in parallel with the staphylococcal preparation.

If the known staphylococcal vaccine Staphypan Berna from the Serum and Vaccine Institute, Bern, Switzerland, is used, a typical treatment schedule may be as follows: eight to ten administrations are made during a period of four to twelve weeks, preferably eight to ten weeks, wherein the dose of the staphylococcal preparation is gradually increased from 0.1 to 1 mL of the pure vaccine. The increase depends on the response from the patient. It may be, for example, 0.1, 0.2, 0.3, 0.4, 0.5, 0.6, 0.7, 0.8, 0.9, and 1.0 mL, respectively. If the patient shows a strong local reaction, it is possible to repeat a dose before increasing it. The dose of staphylococcal preparation in the repeated administration and in maintenance treatment is 1.0 mL.

As described in the published patent, after a pilot study comprising eight patients was made, a double-blind placebo-controlled study was performed, comprising a group of twenty-four women patients fulfilling both the criteria for fibromyalgia and for chronic fatigue syndrome. Seven of the thirteen patients who received the staphylococcal preparation were assessed as being minimally improved, three as being much improved, and the remaining three were unchanged. In the placebo group, three patients were minimally improved, while the remaining eight were unchanged. The improvement in the group with active treatment was statistically significant ($p < 0.05$) compared to the improvement in the placebo group. Following the controlled study, twenty-four patients chose to continue with the treatment and twenty of these have been treated between one and two years. Nineteen of these twenty patients were on the sick list or received sickness pension prior to the start of treatment, and one patient was employed part-time. At a one-year follow-up after the completed study, nine of the twenty patients were in full- or part-time paid employment, while one patient was taking part in a work experience program and one was in the middle of a two-year training program to become a nurse. The treatment strategy used in the above study is a series of administrations of staphylococcal preparations given approximately once a week during a period of some months, for example, three months and thereafter long-term treatment with monthly administrations. Further studies are being conducted by this Swedish group.

STEALTH VIRUS VACCINE

Incomplete forms of herpesviruses may contribute to a newly defined grouping of atypically structured viruses that cause persistent active infection in the absence of significant viral inflammation.[211-213] Designated "stealth viruses," these agents can induce a vacuolating cytopathic effect (CPE) in human and animal cells. The appearance, progression, and wide host range characteristics of the CPE distinguish stealth viruses from conventional human cytopathic viruses, including human herpesviruses, enteroviruses, and adenoviruses. Electron microscopy, serology, and molecular-based assays can be used to further differentiate stealth viruses from conventional viruses.

In published U.S. patent number WO-09960101, W. J. Martin advances the thesis that CFS is but one of many differing manifestations of a persistent stealth viral infection within the brain. Martin states that the involvement of the brain in CFS patients is implied by the historical use of terms such as neurasthenia, myalgic encephalomyelitis, epidemic diencephalomyelitis, and limbic encephalopathy. In more recent years, however, several investigators have argued that the disordered brain function is a secondary phenomenon, resulting, for example, from the overproduction of neuromodulatory cytokines from an activated immune system, that may be responding excessively to a multitude of normally tolerated ubiquitous microorganisms, such as Epstein-Barr virus, human herpesvirus-6, *Candida albicans, Mycoplasma fermentans, Chlamydia pneumoniae,* etc. Attention has also been given to possible brain damage resulting from exposure to environmental neurotoxins, including the potential release into the circulation of neurotoxic bacterial products from a damaged gastrointestinal tract.

Martin goes on to argue that the shift away from a primary infectious process within the brain has occurred in spite of numerous epidemic outbreaks of CFS-like illnesses. Reasons for this neglect include the failure of established CFS investigators to isolate viruses from CFS patients and by the lack of correlation of disease with conventional antiviral serology. Published studies using PCR to test for evidence of retroviruses, enterovirus, and *Mycoplasma* infections were also flawed by erroneous assumptions concerning the specificity of PCR assays when performed under low stringency conditions. The imposition of a restrictive clinical definition of CFS has especially hindered the capacity to validate any suggested new assay, since it required that only patients with fatigue should test positive. This demand has also obscured epidemiological studies for potential disease transmission within families or communities.

Martin described that a stealth virus isolated from a CFS patient induced an acute illness with prominent neurobehavioral changes in cats. Noninflammatory cellular damage was evident in the brain and throughout all of the animal tissues examined. Cellular damage was also present in the offspring of a virus-inoculated pregnant cat. Heat-inactivated virus material did not induce illness when inoculated into a cat. Moreover, this cat did not develop symptoms when subsequently injected with a virus isolated from a different CFS patient. Although stealth viruses may lack antigens required for cellular immunity, they can retain antigens able to evoke circulating antibodies. The presence of stealth virus-reactive antibodies may, in fact, act as a barrier to the bloodborne spread of infection into the brain. The molecular heterogeneity of stealth viruses, however, poses a limitation with using a single antigen for possible immunization.

Immunization designed to elicit protective antibodies can potentially provide protection against an initial infection. The source of antigen can be from a stealth virus or from a conventional virus with antigen structurally related to those on a particular stealth virus isolate.

THIMEROSAL

Thimerosal is a preservative in commercially available influenza virus vaccines (Fluogen, Parke-Davis, Morris Plains, NJ; Fluzone, Connaught Laboratories, Swiftwater, PA; Flu-Immune, Lederle, Wayne, NJ). Studies included in international published patent number WO 98/05350 (Inventor: John McMichael; applicant: Milkhaus Laboratory, Inc., Delanson, New York) provide evidence that thimerosal has antiviral activity and may be useful for the treatment of CFS.

In a first study, a Phase I/II controlled double-blind human clinical trial was conducted using thimerosal-containing compositions for the treatment of chronic fatigue syndrome. Thirty-six patients suffering from documented chronic fatigue syndrome were studied, of whom thirty-three completed the study. Of the subjects who completed the study, seventeen were treated with placebo and sixteen were treated by sublingual administration six times daily of 1 drop (0.05 mL) of a composition comprising 2 μL of influenza vaccine containing 0.01 percent (0.2 μg) thimerosal, 0.4 μL rubella virus vaccine and 576 μL saline. After ten weeks of treatment, the subjects were evaluated and were taken off either drug or placebo and were further evaluated after an additional four weeks of no treatment.

The subjects were evaluated by means of two principle efficacy parameters: a visual analog scale for subjective evaluation of fatigue and a fatigue impact scale comprising thirty-six questions related to cognitive, psychological, and social disorders. Analysis of the results using the visual analog scale showed no statistically significant difference at the 95 percent confidence level between the therapy and the control groups. Although analysis of the results using the fatigue impact scale also failed to demonstrate a statistically significant difference at the 95 percent confidence level between the therapy and placebo groups, the results indicated a trend in favor of the therapy over the placebo indicative of a therapeutic effect.

McMichael went on to perform several experiments and patient treatments with thimerosal-containing fractions of filtrated influenza virus vaccines. Antiherpes activity of thimerosal with and without influenza vaccine was confirmed with in vitro studies and in seven patients. Specifically, a filter centrifugation technique was used to isolate a 30 kD fraction of commercially available influenza virus vaccines (Fluviron and Fluzone), wherein the vaccine was loaded onto an Ultrafree low-binding spin-filter unit with a 30,000 nominal molecular weight limit and centrifuged in a microfuge until all of the fluid had passed through the filter. In vitro assays with the 30 kD filtrate fractions (which contained thimerosal present at a concentration of 0.01 percent as a preservative in the commercial vaccine) saw complete inhibition of herpes virus in a cell culture assay utilizing HSV-1 and HSV-2 infection of A549 (human lung carcinoma) cells.

The fraction obtained was also used in place of dilute influenza virus vaccine in human subjects and was found to improve the clinical response to chronic fatigue syndrome and herpes virus infections. For instance, a fifty-year-old-plus male presented with chronic fatigue syndrome having pronounced lethargy, a history of mental fogginess, and poor quality of life. Two drops of the thimerosal-containing 30 kD influenza virus fraction were administered to the subject sublingually, and the subject reported improvement in excess of 70 percent with an increase in energy and mental clarity for the first time in several years. After three weeks, the subject continued to do well with administration of two drops of the composition daily.

A second double-blind study was carried out on sixteen subjects suffering with chronic fatigue syndrome with three compositions, designated A, B, and C, administered over the course of one month as daily sublingual drops. Each subject was treated by sublingual administration of one drop (0.05 mL) four to six times daily. Composition A comprised 0.0004 percent weight per volume thimerosal (0.2 μg per drop) and 3.2×10^{-7} units neuraminidase per drop in saline. Composition B comprised 0.0004 percent weight per volume thimerosal (0.2 μg per drop) in combination with 0.32 μL rubella virus vaccine (Meruvac, Merck and Co.) in saline. Composition C comprised 0.0004 percent weight per volume thimerosal (0.2 μg per drop) alone in saline. The following parameters were measured by patients' self-reported scores: overall level of fatigue; overall level of pain; severity of flare-ups; muscle cramps; headaches; mental alertness and memory; and overall or average sleep. According to evaluation of these parameters, compositions A and B exhibited significant improvements in the severity of CFS symptoms. Moreover, if the results of one subject treated with composition B are omitted (because physical therapy starting and ending about the same time as the therapy may have adversely affected the results for that subject), the remaining subjects treated with composition B comprising the combination of thimerosal and rubella virus vaccine exhibited the greatest decrease in the severity of chronic fatigue syndrome symptoms.

Preferred dosages of thimerosal for treatment of subjects suffering from herpes virus infections range from about 0.05 μg to 500 μg thimerosal with about 0.5 μg to about 50 μg thimerosal being preferred and about 5 μg thimerosal being particularly preferred. McMichael also isolated a 5 kD fraction from the fluvirin influenza vaccine by further filtration. This fraction, which also contained thimerosal, was effective at inhibiting growth of the herpes virus in the cell culture experiment described above and appeared to be clinically superior in in vivo administration to the 30 kD fraction. The mechanism of action of thimerosal remains to be documented.

TRANSFER FACTORS AGAINST HERPESVIRUSES

Transfer factors (TF) with specific activity against herpesviruses have been documented in CFS. With some studies suggesting that persistent viral activity may play a role in perpetuation of CFS symptoms, there appears to be a rationale for the use of TF in patients with CFS, and some reports have suggested that transfer factors may play a beneficial role in this disorder.[214-217] For instance, specific HHV-6 TF preparation, administered to two CFS patients, inhibited the HHV-6 infection.[215] Prior to treatment, both patients exhibited an activated HHV-6 infection. TF treatment significantly improved the clinical manifestations of CFS in one patient who resumed normal duties within weeks, whereas no clinical improvement was observed in the second patient. Of the twenty patients in a placebo-controlled trial of oral TF,[216] improvement was observed in twelve patients, generally within three to six weeks of beginning treatment. However, in this study, herpes virus serology (EBV and HHV-6) seldom correlated with clinical response. Treatment with TF of a group of 222 patients suffering from cellular immunodeficiency (CID), frequently combined with CFS and/or chronic viral infections by EBV and/or CMV,[217] showed that age but not gender substantially influenced the failure rate of CID treatment using TF. In older people, it is easier to improve the clinical conditions other than CID: this may be related to the diminished number of lymphocytes; however, a placebo effect cannot be totally excluded.

Chapter 4

Concluding Remarks

Recently, researchers have made striking progress in developing therapies for viral disease. The antiviral era is starting to flourish mainly because genomics, the molecular analysis of an organism's entire genetic makeup, has allowed researchers to characterize viral and human genes. This allows scientists to synthesize the proteins that the viruses use to replicate, which in turn opens up avenues for the development of drugs. Previously, it had been impossible to detect and study all but a few such viral proteins. In principle, any step in the viral replicative cycle that differs chemically from normal host cell function can serve as a potential target for the development of antiviral therapy. Moreover, the characterization of the human genetic makeup is helping to unravel many pathways involved in resistance and defenses to viral infections. The ultimate proof of the value of a therapeutic concept is, of course, found only in the clinic or at the bedside, through clinical trials that demonstrate safety and efficacy. Yet genomics can speed up the process immeasurably, and antiviral drugs provide the first glimpse of the era of molecular medicine.

The rapid growth in the number of antiviral medications provides tangible proof that genomics can lead to new and better drugs of all types, whether of natural or synthetic origin. This trend will likely soon lead to new approaches to the treatment of diseases traditionally regarded as nonviral as well as viral diseases. However, there are obstacles that need to be surmounted from side effects to universal accessability of medications and preventive measures. Moreover, appropriate animal models for drug and vaccine testing are crucial to the success of the genomics approach for the discovery of new antivirals and pharmaceuticals of all sorts. The lack of such models for many diseases, including chronic fatigue syndrome, is proving to be a major bottleneck for the pharmaceutical industry, academia, and public sector efforts.

Still, the future looks bright, and patients with chronic fatigue syndrome have a broader spectrum of therapeutic choices. Also, the categorization of CFS patients according to prevailing symptomatology is helping to better target particular disease manifestations and to design clinical trials where findings are not diluted against a background of patient heterogeneity, which stems from a diverse range of circumstances from natural disease progression and exacerbation-remission cycles to prevailing symptomatology at the time of assessment. It is the hope of the author that this book will serve as inspiration for further research in this area.

Notes

1. Osterholm MT. Emerging infections—Another warning. *The New England Journal of Medicine* 342(17):1280-1281, 2000.

2. Frothingham C. The relation between acute infectious diseases and arterial lesions. *Archives of Internal Medicine* 8:153-162, 1911.

3. Ophüls W. Arteriosclerosis and cardiovascular disease: Their relation to infectious diseases. *Journal of the American Medical Association* 76:700-701, 1921.

4. Fabricant CG, Fabricant J, Litrenta MM, Minick CR. Virus-induced atherosclerosis. *Journal of Experimental Medicine* 148:335-340, 1978.

5. Danesh J, Collins R, Peto R. Chronic infections and coronary heart disease: Is there a link? *Lancet* 350:430-436, 1997.

6. Buja LM. Does atherosclerosis have an infectious etiology? *Circulation* 94:872-873, 1996.

7. Libby P, Egan D, Skarlatos S. Roles of infectious agents in atherosclerosis and restenosis: An assessment of the evidence and need for future research. *Circulation* 96:4095-4103, 1997.

8. Kullo IJ, Gau GT, Tajik J. Novel risk factors for atherosclerosis. *Mayo Clinic Proceedings* 75:369-380, 2000.

9. Benitez M. Atherosclerosis: An infectious disease? *Hospital Practice,* September 1, 1999.

10. Talal N, Dauphinée MJ, Dang H, Alexander SS, Hart DJ, Garry RF. Detection of serum antibodies to retroviral proteins in patients with primary Sjögren's syndrome (autoimmune exocrinopathy). *Arthritis and Rheumatism* 33(6):774-781, 1990.

11. Talal N, Garry RF, Schur PH, Alexander S, Dauphinée MJ, Livas IH, Ballester A, Takei M, Dang H. A conserved idiotype and antibodies to retroviral proteins in systemic lupus erythematosus. *Journal of Clinical Investigation* 85(6):1866-1887, 1990.

12. Perl A, Gorevic PD, Condemi JJ, Papsidero L, Poiesz BJ, Abraham GN. Antibodies to retroviral proteins and reverse transcriptase activity in patients with essential cryoglobulinemia. *Arthritis and Rheumatism* 34(10):313-318, 1991.

13. Dang H, Dauphinée MJ, Talal N, Garry RF, Seibold JR, Medsger TA Jr, Alexander S, Feghali CA. Serum antibody to retroviral gag proteins in systemic sclerosis. *Arthritis and Rheumatism* 34(10):1336-1337, 1991.

14. Garry RF, Fermin CD, Hart DJ, Alexander SS, Donehower LA, Luo-Zhang H. Detection of a human intracisternal A-type retroviral particle antigenically related to HIV. *Science* 250(4894):1127-1129, 1990.

15. Banki K, Maceda J, Hurley E, Ablonczy E, Mattson DH, Szegedy L, Hung C, Perl A. Human T-cell lymphotropic virus (HTLV)-related endogenous sequence, HRES-1, encodes a 28-kDa protein: A possible autoantigen for HTLV-I gag reactive autoantibodies. *Proceedings of the National Academy of Sciences USA* 89(5):1939-1943, 1992.

16. Blick M, Bresser J, Lepe-Zuniga JL, Goodacre A, Luethke D, Holder WR, Duvic M. Identification of human immunodeficiency virus hybridizing sequences in the peripheral blood of a patient with systemic lupus erythematosus. *Journal of the American Academy of Dermatology* 23(4 Part 1):641-645, 1990.

17. Ciampolillo A, Marini V, Mirakian R, Buscema M, Schulz T, Pujol-Borrel R, Bottazzo GF. Retrovirus-like sequences in Graves disease: Implications for human autoimmunity. *Lancet* 1(8647):1096-110, 1989.

18. Lagaye S, Vexiau P, Morozov V, Guenebaut-Claudet V, Tobaly-Tapiero J, Canivet M, Cathelineau G, Peries J, Emanoil-Ravier R. Human spumaretrovirus-related sequences in the DNA of leukocytes from patients with Graves disease. *Proceedings of the National Academy of Sciences USA* 89(21):10070-10074, 1992.

19. Silvestris F, Williams RC, Dammacco F. Autoreactivity in HIV-1 infection: The role of molecular mimicry. *Clinical Immunology and Immunopathology* 75:197-205, 1995.

20. Atkinson MA, Bowman MA, Campbell L, Darrow BL, Kaufman DL, Maclaren NK. Cellular immunity to a determinant common in glutamate decarboxylase and coxsackievirus in insulin-dependent diabetes. *Journal of Clinical Investigation* 94(5):2125-2129, 1994.

21. Tian J, Lehmann PV, Kaufman DL. T cell cross-reactivity between coxsackievirus and glutamate decarboxylase is associated with a murine diabetes susceptibility allele. *Journal of Experimental Medicine* 180:1979-1984, 1994.

22. Jones DB, Armstrong NW. Coxsackievirus and diabetes revisited. *Nature Medicine* 1:284, 1995.

23. Trujillo JR, McLane MF, Lee T-H, Essex M. Molecular mimicry between the human immunodeficiency virus type 1 gp120 V3 loop and human brain proteins. *Journal of Virology* 67:7711-7715, 1993.

24. Gama Sosa MA, De Gasperi R, Patarca R, Fletcher MA, Kolodny EH. Antisulfatide IgG antibodies recognize HIV proteins. *Journal of Acquired Immune Deficiency Syndromes and Human Retrovirology* 15:83-90, 1997.

25. Holmes GP, Kaplan JE, Gantz NM, Komaroff AL, Schonberger LB, Straus SE, Jones JF, Dubois RE, Cunningham-Rundles C, Pahwa S, et al.

Chronic fatigue syndrome: A working case definition. *Annals of Internal Medicine* 108(3):387-389, 1988.

26. Klimas NG, Fletcher MA. Chronic fatigue syndrome. *Current Opinion in Infectious Diseases* 8:145-148, 1995.

27. Buchwald D, Cheney PR, Peterson DL, Henry B, Wormsley SB, Geiger A, Ablashi DV, Salahuddin SZ, Saxinger C, Biddle R, et al. A chronic illness characterized by fatigue, neurologic and immunologic disorders and active human herpesvirus 6 type infection. *Annals of Internal Medicine* 116(2):103-113, 1992.

28. Millon C, Salvato F, Blaney F, Morgan R, Mantero-Atienza E, Klimas NG, Fletcher MA. A psychological assessment of chronic fatigue syndrome/chronic Epstein-Barr virus patients. *Psychology and Health* 3:131-141, 1989.

29. Lutgendorf S, Klimas N, Antoni M, Brickman A, Fletcher MA. Relationships of cognitive difficulties, depression and illness burden in chronic fatigue syndrome. *Journal of Chronic Fatigue Syndrome* 1:23-41, 1995.

30. Fukuda K, Straus SE, Hickie I, Sharpe MC, Dobbins JG, Komaroff A, International CFS Study Group. The chronic fatigue syndrome: A comprehensive approach to its definition and study. *Annals of Internal Medicine* 121:953-959, 1994.

31. Patarca R. *Concise Encyclopedia of Chronic Fatigue Syndrome.* The Haworth Press Inc., Binghamton, NY, pp. 1 ff, 2000.

32. Klimas NG, Morgan R, Salvato F, van Riel F, Millon C, Fletcher MA. Chronic fatigue syndrome and psychoneuroimmunology. In *Stress and Disease Progression: Perspectives in Behavioral Medicine.* Schneiderman N, McCabe P, Baum A, Eds. Lawrence Erlbaum, Assoc., Hillsdale, NJ, pp. 121-137, 1992.

33. Chester AC, Levine PH. Concurrent sick building syndrome and chronic fatigue syndrome. *Clinical Infectious Diseases* 18(suppl. 1):S43-S48, 1994.

34. Ablashi DV, Kramarsky B, Bernbaum J, Whitman JE, Pearson GR. Viruses and chronic fatigue syndrome: Current status. *Journal of Chronic Fatigue Syndrome* 1:3-22, 1995.

35. Lederberg J. Infectious history. *Science* 288:287-293, 2000.

36. St. George IM. Did Cook's sailors have Tapanui flu? Chronic fatigue syndrome on the resolution. *New Zealand Medical Journal* 109(1014):15-17, 1996.

37. Lindal E, Bergmann S, Thorlacius S, Stefansson JG. Anxiety disorders: A result of long-term chronic fatigue—The psychiatric characteristics of the sufferers of Iceland disease. *Acta Neurologica Scandinavica* 96(3):158-162, 1997.

38. Marwick C. International plan focuses on eradication of polio and containment of the virus. *Journal of the American Medical Association* 283(12):1553-1554, 2000.

39. Josephs SF, Wong-Staal F, Manzari V, Gallo RC, Sodroski JG, Trus M, Perkins D, Patarca R, Haseltine WA. Long terminal repeat structure of an American isolate of type I human T-cell leukemia virus. *Virology* 139:340-345, 1984.

40. Sodroski J, Trus M, Perkins D, Patarca R, Wong-Staal F, Gelman E, Gallo RC, Haseltine WA. Repetitive structure in the long terminal repeat element of a type II human T-cell leukemia virus. *Proceedings of the National Academy of Sciences USA* 81:4617-4621, 1984.

41. Sodroski J, Patarca R, Perkins D, Briggs D, Lee T, Essex M, Colligan J, Wong-Staal F, Gallo RC, Haseltine WA. Sequence of the envelope glycoprotein gene of type II human T-lymphotropic virus. *Science* 225:421-423, 1984.

42. Haseltine WA, Sodroski JG, Patarca R, Briggs D, Perkins D, Wong-Staal F. Structure of the 3'-terminal region of type II human T-lymphotropic virus: Evidence for a new coding region. *Science* 225:419-421, 1984.

43. Ratner L, Haseltine WA, Patarca R, Livak K, Starcich B, Josephs SF, Doran ER, Rafalski JA, Whitehorn EA, Baumeister K, Ivanoff L, Petterway SR, Pearson ML, Lautenberger JA, Papas TS, Ghrayeb J, Chang NT, Gallo RC, Wong-Staal F. Complete nucleotide sequence of the AIDS virus, HTLV-III. *Nature* 313:277-284, 1985.

44. Sodroski J, Patarca R, Rosen C, Wong-Staal F, Haseltine WA. Location of the *trans*-activating region on the genome of human T-cell lymphotropic virus type III. *Science* 229:74-77, 1985.

45. Patarca R, Heath C, Goldenberg GJ, Rosen CA, Sodroski JG, Haseltine WA, Hansen UM. In vitro transcription directed by the HIV LTR. *AIDS Research and Human Retroviruses* 3:41-56, 1987.

46. Patarca R, Dorta B, Ramirez JL. Creation of a database for sequences of ribosomal nucleic acids and detection of conserved restriction endonucleases sites through computerized processing. *Nucleic Acids Research* 10(1):175-182, 1982.

47. Patarca R, Haseltine WA. Sequence similarity among retroviruses. *Nature* 309:728, 1984.

48. Patarca R, Haseltine WA. Similarities among retrovirus proteins. *Nature* 312:496, 1984.

49. Patarca R, Haseltine WA. A major retroviral core protein related to EPA and TIMP. *Nature* 318:390, 1985.

50. Patarca R, Haseltine WA. Variation among the human T-lymphotropic virus type III (HTLV-III/LAV) strains. *Journal of Theoretical Biology* 125:213-217, 1986.

51. Patarca R, Haseltine WA. Letter to the editor. *AIDS Research and Human Retroviruses* 3:1-2, 1987.

52. Elfassi E, Patarca R, Haseltine WA. Similarities among the pre-S regions of hepatitis B viruses: Analogy with retroviral transmembrane proteins. *Journal of Theoretical Biology* 121:371-374, 1986.

53. Haseltine WA, Patarca R. AIDS virus and scrapie agent share protein. *Nature* 323:115-116, 1986.

54. Patarca R, Haseltine WA, Webster T, Smith TF. Of how great significance. *Nature* 326:749, 1987.

55. Webster T, Patarca R, Lathrop R, Smith TF. Potential structural motifs for reverse transcriptases. *Molecular Biology and Evolution* 6:317-320, 1989.

56. Mitsuya H, Broder S. Strategies for antiviral therapy in AIDS. *Nature* 325:773-778, 1987.

57. Mitsuya H, Yarchoan R, Broder S. Molecular targets for AIDS therapy. *Science* 249:1533-1544, 1990.

58. Yarchoan R, Pluda JM, Perno CF, Mitsuya H, Broder S. Antiretroviral therapy of human immunodeficiency virus infection: Current strategies and challenges for the future. *Blood* 78(4):859-884, 1991.

59. Hirsch MS, Kaplan JC. Treatment of human immunodeficiency virus infections. *Antimicrobial Agents and Chemotherapy* 31:839-843, 1987.

60. Johnson MI, Hoth DF. Present status and future prospects for HIV therapies. *Science* 260:1286-1293, 1993.

61. De Clercq E. Antiviral therapy for human immunodeficiency virus infections. *Clinical Microbiology Reviews* 8:200-239, 1995.

62. De Clercq E. In search of a selective antiviral chemotherapy. *Clinical Microbiology Reviews* 10:674-693, 1997.

63. Erickson JW, Fesik SW. Macromolecular X-ray crystallography and NM as tools for structure-based drug design. *Annual Review of Medicinal Chemistry* 27:271-289, 1992.

64. Robins RK. Synthetic antiviral agents. *Chemical Engineering News,* January 27:28-40, 1986.

65. Tummino PJ, Prasad JVNV, Ferguson D, Nouhan C, Graham N, Dormagala JM, Ellsworth E, Gajda C, Hagen SE, Lunney EA, Parak S, Tait BD, Pavlovsky A, Erickson JW, Gracheck S, McQuade TJ, Hupe DJ. Discovery and optimization of nonpeptide HIV-1 protease inhibitors. *Bioorganic Medicine Chemistry Letters* 4(9):1401-1410, 1996.

66. Erickson J, Neidhart DJ, Van Dri J, Kempf DJ, Wang XC, Norbeck DW, Plattner JJ, Rittenhouse JW, Turon M, Wideburg N, et al. Design, activity, and 2.8 A crystal structure of C_2 symmetric inhibitor complexed to HIV-1 protease. *Science* 249(4968):527-533, 1990.

67. Wlodawer A, Erickson JW. Structure-based inhibitors of HIV-1 protease. *Annual Reviews of Biochemistry* 62:543-585, 1993.

68. Esparza J. The role of United Nations HIV/AIDS Program (UNAIDS) in the prevention of the viral transmission. *Medicina* 58:69-70, 1998.

69. McCune JM, Namikawa R, Shih C-C, Robin L, Kaneshima H. Suppression of HIV infection in AZT-treated SCID-hu mice. *Science* 247(4942):564-566, 1990.

70. Mosier DE, Gulizia RJ, Baird SM, Wilson DB, Spector DH, Spector SA. Human immunodeficiency virus infection of human PBL-SCID mice. *Science* 251(4995):791-794, 1991.

71. Koff WC, Elm JL Jr, Halstead SB. Antiviral effects of ribavirin and 6-mercapto-9-tetrahydro-2-furylpurine against dengue viruses in vitro. *Antiviral Research* 2(1-2):69-79, 1982.

72. De Vincenzo J. Prevention and treatment of respiratory syncytial virus infections. *Advances in Pediatric Infectious Diseases* 13:1-47, 1997.

73. Gubareva LV, Kaiser L, Hayden FG. Influenza virus neuraminidase inhibitor. *Lancet* 355:827-835, 2000.

74. Monto AS, Fleming DM, Henry D, de Groot R, Makela M, Klein T, Elliott M, Keene ON, Man CY. Efficacy and safety of the neuraminidase inhibitor zanamivir in the treatment of influenza A and B virus infections. *Journal of Infectious Diseases* 180(2):256-261, 1999.

75. Blaser MJ. The changing relationships of *Helicobacter pylori* and humans: Implications for health and disease. *Journal of Infectious Diseases* 179:1523-1530, 1999.

76. Hadley SK, Petry JJ. Medicinal herbs: A primer for primary care. *Hospital Practice* 34(6):105-123, 1999.

77. Fohlman J, Friman G, Tuvemo T. Enterovirus infections in new disguise. *Lakartidningen* 94(28-29):2555-2560, 1997.

78. Galbraith DN, Nairn C, Clements GB. Evidence for enteroviral persistence in humans. *Journal of General Virology* 78 (Pt 2):307-312, 1997.

79. Hill WM. Are echoviruses still orphan? *British Journal of Biomedical Sciences* 53(3):221-226, 1996.

80. Archard LC, Bowles NE, Behan PO, Bell EJ, Doyle D. Post viral fatigue syndrome: Persistence of enterovirus RNA in muscle and elevated creatinine kinase. *Journal of the Royal Society of Medicine* 81:326-329, 1988.

81. Miller NA, Carmichael, HA, Hall FC, Calder BD. Antibody to Coxsackie B virus in diagnosing postviral fatigue syndrome. *British Medical Journal* 302:140-143, 1991.

82. Buchwald D, Ashley RL, Pearlman T, Kith P, Komaroff AL. Viral serologies in patients with chronic fatigue and chronic fatigue syndrome. *Journal of Medical Virology* 50(1):25-30, 1996.

83. Lindh G, Samuelson A, Hedlund KO, Evengard B, Lindquist L, Ehrnst A. No findings of enteroviruses in Swedish patients with chronic fa-

tigue syndrome. *Scandinavian Journal of Infectious Diseases* 28(3):305-307, 1996.

84. McArdle A, McArdle F, Jackson MJ, Page SF, Fahal I, Edwards RH. Investigation by polymerase chain reaction of enteroviral infection in patients with chronic fatigue syndrome. *Clinical Science* 90(4):295-300, 1996.

85. Glaser R, Kiecolt-Glaser JK. Stress-associated immune modulation: Relevance to viral infections and chronic fatigue syndrome. *American Journal of Medicine* 105(3A):35S-42S, 1998.

86. Jones JF, Ray CG, Minnich LL, Hick MJ, Kibler R, Lucus DO. Evidence for active Epstein-Barr virus infection in patients with persistent unexplained illnesses; elevated anti-early antigen antibodies. *Annals of Internal Medicine* 102:1-7, 1985.

87. Hellinger WC, Smith TF, Van Scoy RE, Spidzor PG, Forgacs P, Edson RS. Chronic fatigue syndrome and diagnostic utility of antibody to Epstein-Barr virus early antigen. *Journal of the American Medical Association* 260:971-973, 1988.

88. Bennett BK, Hickie IB, Vollmer-Conna US, Quigley B, Brennan CM, Wakefield D, Douglas MP, Hansen GR, Tahmindjis AJ, Lloyd AR. The relationship between fatigue, psychological and immunological variables in acute infectious illness. *Australia and New Zealand Journal of Psychiatry* 32(2):180-186, 1998.

89. White PD, Thomas JM, Amess J, Crawford DH, Grover SA, Kangro HO, Clare AW. Incidence, risk and prognosis of acute and chronic fatigue syndromes and psychiatric disorders after glandular fever. *British Journal of Psychiatry* 173:475-481, 1998.

90. Schmaling KB, Jones JF. MMPI profiles of patients with chronic fatigue syndrome. *Journal of Psychosomatic Research* 40(1):67-74, 1996.

91. Buchwald D, Ashley RL, Pearlman T, Kith P, Komaroff AL. Viral serologies in patients with chronic fatigue and chronic fatigue syndrome. *Journal of Medical Virology* 50(1):25-30, 1996.

92. Braun DK, Dominguez G, Pellett PE. Human herpesvirus 6. *Clinical Microbiology Reviews* 10(3):521-567, 1997.

93. Marsh S, Kaplan M, Asano Y, Hoekzema D, Komaroff AL, Whitman JE Jr, Ablashi DV. Development and application of HHV-6 antigen capture assay for the detection of HHV-6 infections. *Journal of Virological Methods* 61(1-2):103-112, 1996.

94. Cuende JI, Civeira P, Diez N, Prieto J. High prevalence without reactivation of herpes virus 6 in subjects with chronic fatigue syndrome. *Anales de Medicina Interna* 14(9):441-444, 1997.

95. Levy JA, Greenspan D, Ferro F, Lennette ET. Frequent isolation of HHV-6 from saliva and high seroprevalence of the virus in the population. *Lancet* 335:1047-1050, 1990.

96. Ablashi DV, Handy M, Bernbaum J, Chatlynne LG, Lapps W, Kramarsky B, Berneman ZN, Komaroff AL, Whitman JE. Propagation and characterization of human herpesvirus-7 (HHV-7) isolates in a continuous T-lymphoblastoid cell line (SUPT1). *Journal of Virological Methods* 73(2):123-140, 1998.

97. Martin WJ. Cellular sequences in stealth viruses. *Pathobiology* 66(2):53-58, 1998.

98. Martin WJ. Detection of RNA sequences in cultures of a stealth virus isolated form the cerebrospinal fluid of a health care worker with chronic fatigue syndrome. Case report. *Pathobiology* 65(1):57-60, 1997.

99. Martin WJ. Severe stealth virus encephalopathy following chronic-fatigue-syndrome-like illness: Clinical and histopathological features. *Pathobiology* 64(1):1-8, 1996.

100. Martin WJ. Genetic instability and fragmentation of a stealth viral genome. *Pathobiology* 64(1):9-17, 1996.

101. Gunn W, Komaroff A, Levine S, Connell D, Multilab retrovirus test results for CFS patients from three different geographical areas. *Mortality and Morbidity Weekly Report* pp. 1ff., 1997.

102. DeFreitas E, Hilliand B, Cheney P, Bell D, Kiggundu E, Sankey D, Wroblewska Z, Palladino M, Woodward JP, Koprowski H. Retroviral sequences related to human T-lymphotropic virus type II in patients with chronic fatigue immune dysfunction syndrome. *Proceedings of the National Academy of Sciences USA* 88(7):2922-2926, 1991.

103. Holmes MJ, Diack DS, Easingwood A, Cross JP, Carlisle B. Electron microscope immunocytological profiles in chronic fatigue syndrome. *Journal of Psychiatric Research* 31(1):115-122, 1997.

104. Jacobson SK, Daly JS, Thorne GM, McIntosh K. Chronic parvovirus B19 infection resulting in chronic fatigue syndrome: Case history and review. *Clinical Infectious Diseases* 24(6):1048-1051, 1997.

105. Bennett BK, Hickie IB, Vollmer-Conna US, Quigley B, Brennan CM, Wakefield D, Douglas MP, Hansen GR, Tahmindjis AJ, Lloyd AR. The relationship between fatigue, psychological and immunological variables in acute infectious illness. *Australia and New Zealand Journal of Psychiatry* 32(2):180-186, 1998.

106. Stitz L, Bilzer T, Tich JA, Rott R. Pathogenesis of Borna disease. *Archives of Virology* 7:135-151, 1993.

107. Bode L, Fersyt R, Czech G. Borna disease virus infection and affective disorders in man. *Archives of Virology* 7:159-167, 1993.

108. Sauder C, Muller A, Cubitt B, Mayer J, Steimetz J, Trabert W, Ziegler B, Wanke K, Mueller-Lantzsch N, de la Torre JC, Grasser FA. Detection of Borna disease virus (BDV) antibodies and BDV RNA psychiatric patients: Evidence of high sequence conservation of human blood-derived RNA. *Journal of Virology* 70(1):7713-7724, 1996.

109. Salvatore M, Morozunov M, Schnemake M, Lipkin WI, and the Bornavirus study group. Borna disease virus in brains of North American and European people with schizophrenia and bipolar disorders. *Lancet* 349:1813-1814, 1998.

110. Nakaya T, Kuratsune H, Kitani T, Ikuta K. Demonstration on Borna disease virus in patients with chronic fatigue syndrome. *Nippon Rinsho—Japanese Journal of Clinical Medicine* 55(11):3064-3071, 1997.

111. Kitani T, Kuratsune H, Fuke I, Nakamura Y, Nakaya T, Asahi S, Tobiume M, Yamaguti M, Machii T, Inagi R, Yamanishi K, Ikuta K. Possible correlation between Borna disease virus infection and Japanese patients with chronic fatigue syndrome. *Microbiology and Immunology* 40(6):459-462, 1996.

112. Nakaya T, Takahashi H, Nakamura Y, Asahi S, Tobiume M, Kuratsune H, Kitani T, Yamanishi K, Ikuta K. Demonstration of Borna disease virus RNA in peripheral blood mononuclear cells derived from Japanese patients with chronic fatigue syndrome. *FEBS Letters* 378(2):145-149, 1996.

113. Levine S. Borna disease virus proteins in patients with CFS. *Journal of Chronic Fatigue Syndrome* 5(3/4):199-206, 1999.

114. Konstantinov K, von Mikecz A, Buchwald D, Jones J, Gerace L, Tan EM. Autoantibodies to nuclear antigens in chronic fatigue syndrome. *Journal of Clinical Investigation* 98(8):1888-1896, 1996.

115. Poteliakhoff A. Fatigue syndromes and the aetiology of autoimmune disease. *Journal of Chronic Fatigue Syndrome* 4(4):31-50, 1998.

116. von Mikecz A, Konstantinov K, Buchwald DS, Gerace L, Tan EM. High frequency of autoantibodies in patients with chronic fatigue syndrome. *Arthritis and Rheumatism* 40(2):295-305, 1997.

117. Keller RH, Lane JL, Klimas N, Reiter WM, Fletcher MA, van Riel F, Morgan R. Association between HLA class II antigens and the chronic fatigue immune dysfunction syndrome. *Clinical Infectious Diseases* 18(Suppl 1):S154-S156, 1994.

118. Jones J. Serologic and immunologic responses in chronic fatigue syndrome with emphasis on the Epstein-Barr virus. *Reviews of Infectious Diseases* 13(1):S26-S31, 1991.

119. Jones JF, Straus SE. Chronic Epstein-Barr virus infection. *Annual Reviews of Medicine* 38:195-209, 1987.

120. Jones JF, Ray G, Minnich LL, Hicks MJ, Kibler R, Lucas DO. Evidence for active Epstein-Barr virus infection in patients with persistent, unexplained illnesses: Elevated anti-early antigen antibodies. *Annals of Internal Medicine* 102(1):1-7, 1985.

121. Kaslow JE, Rucker L, Onishi R. Liver extract-folic acid-cyanocobalamin vs. placebo for chronic fatigue syndrome. *Archives of Internal Medicine* 149:2501-2503, 1989.

122. Prieto J, Subira ML, Castilla A, Serrano M. Naloxone-reversible monocyte dysfunction in patients with chronic fatigue syndrome. *Scandinavian Journal of Immunology* 30(1):13-20, 1989.

123. Salit IE. Sporadic postinfectious neuromyasthenia. *Canadian Medical Association Journal* 133:659-663, 1985.

124. Straus SE, Tosato G, Armstrong G, Lawley T, Preble OT, Henle W, Davey R, Pearson G, Epstein J, Brus I, et al. Persisting illness and fatigue in adults with evidence of Epstein-Barr virus infection. *Annals of Internal Medicine* 102(1):7-16, 1985.

125. Tobi M, Morag A, Ravid Z, Chowers I, Feldman-Weiss V, Michaeli Y, Ben-Chetrit E, Shalit M, Knobler H. Prolonged atypical illness associated with serological evidence of persistent Epstein-Barr infection. *Lancet* 1(8263):61-64, 1982.

126. Bates DW, Buchwald D, Lee J, Kith P, Doolittle T, Rutherford C, Churchill WH, Schur PH, Werner M, Wybenga D, et al. Clinical laboratory test findings in patients with chronic fatigue syndrome. *Archives of Internal Medicine* 155(1):97-103, 1995.

127. Gold D, Bowden R, Sixbey J, Riggs R, Katon WJ, Ashley R, Obrigewitch RM, Corey L. Chronic fatigue. A prospective clinical and virologic study. *Journal of the American Medical Association* 264(1):48-53, 1990.

128. Behan PO, Behan WHM, Bell EJ. The postviral fatigue syndrome—An analysis of the findings in 50 cases. *Journal of Infectious Diseases* 10:211-222, 1985.

129. Weinstein L. Thyroiditis and "chronic infectious mononucleosis." *New England Journal of Medicine* 317:1225-1226, 1987.

130. Plioplys AV. Antimuscle and anti-CNS circulating antibodies in chronic fatigue syndrome. *Neurology* 48(6):1717-1719, 1997.

131. Rasmussen AK, Nielsen AH, Andersen V, Barington T, Bendtzen K, Hansen MB, Nielsen L, Pederson BK, Wiik A. Chronic fatigue syndrome—A controlled cross sectional study. *Journal of Rheumatology* 21(8):1527-1531, 1994.

132. Itoh Y, Hamada H, Imai T, Saki T, Igarashi T, Yuge K, Fukunaga Y, Yamamoto M. Antinuclear antibodies in children with chronic nonspecific complaints. *Autoimmunity* 25(4):243-250, 1997.

133. Fiore G, Giacovazzo F, Giacovazzo M. Three cases of dermatomyositis erroneously diagnosed as "chronic fatigue syndrome." *European Reviews of Medical and Pharmacological Sciences* 1(6):193-195, 1997.

134. Nishikai M, Akiya K, Tojo T, Onoda N, Tani M, Shimizu K. "Seronegative" Sjoegren's syndrome manifested as a subset of chronic fatigue syndrome. *British Journal of Rheumatology* 35(5):471-474, 1996.

135. Barendregt PJ, Visser MR, Smets EM, Tulen JH, van den Meiracker AH, Boomsma F, Markusse HM. Fatigue in primary Sjogren's syndrome. *Annals of Rheumatic Diseases* 57(5):291-295, 1998.

136. Asim M, Turney JH. The female patient with faints and fatigue: Don't forget Sjogren's syndrome. *Nephrology, Dialysis, Transplantation* 12(7):1516-1517, 1997.

137. Wang B, Gladman DD, Urowitz MB. Fatigue in lupus is not correlated with disease activity. *Journal of Rheumatology* 25(5):892-895, 1998.

138. Jones SD, Koh WH, Steiner A, Garrett SL, Calin A. Fatigue in ankylosing spondylitis: Its prevalence and relationship to disease activity, sleep, and other factors. *Journal of Rheumatology* 23(3):487-490, 1996.

139. Wolfe F, Hawley DJ, Wilson K. The prevalence and meaning of fatigue in rheumatic disease. *Journal of Rheumatology* 23(8):1407-1417, 1996.

140. Huyser BA, Parker JC, Thoreson R, Smarr KL, Johnson JC, Hoffman R. Predictors of subjective fatigue among individuals with rheumatoid arthritis. *Arthritis and Rheumatism* 41(12):2230-2237, 1998.

141. Riemsma RP, Rasker JJ, Taal E, Griep EN, Wouters JM, Wiegman O. Fatigue in rheumatoid arthritis: The role of self-efficacy and problematic social support. *British Journal of Rheumatology* 37(10):1042-1046, 1998.

142. Stone AA, Broderick JE, Porter LS, Kaell AT. The experience of rheumatoid arthritis pain and fatigue: Examining momentary reports and correlates over one week. *Arthritis Care and Research* 10(3):185-193, 1997.

143. Shaheen SO, Aaby P, Hall AJ, Barker DJ, Heyes CB, Shiell AW, Goudiaby A. Measles and atopy in Guinea-Bissau. *Lancet* 347:1792-1796, 1996.

144. Aaby P. Assumptions and contradictions in measles and measles immunization research: Is measles good for something? *Social Sciences Medicine* 41(5):673-686, 1995.

145. Aaby P, Samb B, Simondon F, Seck AM, Knudsen K, Whittle H. Non-specific beneficial effect of measles immunisation: Analysis of mortality studies from developing countries. *British Medical Journal* 311(7003):481-485, 1995.

146. Mu HH, Sewell WA. Enhancement of interleukin-4 production by pertussis toxin. *Infection and Immunity* 61(7):3190-3198, 1993.

147. Ramiya VK, Shang XZ, Pharis PG, Wasserfall CH, Stabler TV, Muir AB, Schatz DA, Maclaren NK. Antigen-based therapies to prevent diabetes in NOD mice. *Journal of Autoimmunity* 9:349-356, 1996.

148. Smit JA, Stark JH, Myburgh JA. Induction of primate TH2 lymphokines to suppress TH1 cells. *Transplantation Proceedings* 28(2):665-666, 1996.

149. Nilsson L, Kjellman NI, Storsaeter J, Gustafsson L, Olin P. Lack of association between pertussis vaccine and symptoms of asthma and allergy. *Journal of the American Medical Association* 275(10):760, 1996.

150. Odent MR, Culpin EE, Kimmel T. Pertussis vaccination and asthma: Is there a link? *Journal of the American Medical Association* 272(8):592-593, 1994.

151. Bretscher PA, Wei G, Menon JN, Bielefeldt-Ohmann H. Establishment of stable, cell-mediated immunity that makes "susceptible" mice resistant to *Leishmania major. Science* 257(5069):539-542, 1992.

152. Hernandez-Pando R, Rook GA. The role of TNF-alpha in T-cell mediated inflammation depends on the Th1/Th2 cytokine balance. *Immunology* 82(4):591-595, 1994.

153. Bernton E, Hoover D, Galloway R, Popp K. Adaptation to chronic stress in military trainees. Adrenal androgens, testosterone, glucocorticoids, IGF-1, and immune function. *Annals of the New York Academy of Sciences* 774:217-231, 1995.

154. Brinkmann V, Kristofic C. Regulation of corticosteroids of Th1 and Th2 cytokine production in human CD4+ effector T cells generated from CD45RO- and CD45RO+ subsets. *Journal of Immunology* 155(7):3322-3328, 1995.

155. Ramirez F, Fowell DJ, Puklavee M, Simmonds S, Mason D. Glucocorticoids promote a Th2 cytokine response by CD4+ T cells in vitro. *Journal of Immunology* 156(7): 2406-2412, 1996.

156. Daynes RA, Araneo BA, Ershler WB, Maloney C, Li GZ, Ryu SY. Altered regulation of IL-6 production with normal aging. Possible linkage to the age-associated decline in dehydroepiandrosterone and its sulfated derivative. *Journal of Immunology* 150(12):5219-5230, 1993.

157. Garg M, Bondade S. Reversal of age-associated decline in immune response to Pnu-immune vaccine by supplementation with the steroid hormone dehydroepiandrosterone. *Infection and Immunity* 61(5):2238-2241, 1993.

158. Morales AJ, Nolan JJ, Nelson JC, Yen SS. Effects of replacement dose of dehydroepiandrosterone in men and women of advancing age. *Journal of Clinical Endocrinology and Metabolism* 78(6):1360-1367, 1994.

159. Daynes RA, Araneo BA. Contrasting effects of glucocorticoids on the capacity of T cells to produce the growth factors interleukin 2 and interleukin 4. *European Journal of Immunology* 19(12):2319-2325, 1989.

160. Daynes RA, Araneo BA, Dowell TA, Huang K, Dudley D. Regulation of murine lymphokine production in vivo. III. The lymphoid tissue microenvironment exerts regulatory influences over T helper cell function. *Journal of Experimental Medicine* 171(4):979-996, 1990.

161. Daynes RA, Araneo BA, Hennebold J, Enioutina E, Mu HH. Steroids as regulators of the mammalian immune response. *Journal of Investigative Dermatology* 105:14S-19S, 1995.

162. Daynes RA, Meikle AW, Araneo BA. Locally active steroid hormones may facilitate compartmentalization of immunity by regulating the types of lymphokines produced by helper T cells. *Research in Immunology* 142(1):40-45, 1991.

163. Suzuki T, Suzuki N, Daynes RA, Engleman EG. Dehydroepiandrosterone enhances IL2 production and cytotoxic effector function of human T cells. *Clinical Immunology and Immunopathology* 61(2):202-211, 1991.

164. Fischer A, Konig W. Influence of cytokines and cellular interactions on the glucocorticoid-induced Ig (E, G, A, M) synthesis of peripheral blood mononuclear cells. *Immunology* 74(2):228-233, 1991.

165. Guida L, O'Hehir RE, Hawrylowicz CM. Synergy between dexamethasone and interleukin-5 for the induction of major histocompatibility complex class II expression by human peripheral blood eosinophils. *Blood* 84(8):2733-2740, 1994.

166. Padgett DA, Sheridan JF, Loria RM. Steroid hormone regulation of a polyclonal TH2 immune response. *Annals of the New York Academy of Sciences* 774:323-325, 1995.

167. Wu CY, Sarfati M, Heusser C, Fournier S, Rubio-Trujillo M, Peleman R, Delespesse G. Glucocorticoids increase the synthesis of immunoglobulin E by interleukin 4-stimulated human lymphocytes. *Journal of Clinical Investigation* 87(3):870-877, 1991.

168. Corrigan CJ, Hamid Q, North J, Barkans J, Moqbel R, Durham S, Gemou-Engesaeth V, Kay AB. Peripheral blood CD4 but not CD8 T-lymphocytes in patients with exacerbation of asthma transcribe and translate messenger RNA encoding cytokines which prolong eosinophil survival in the context of a Th2-type pattern: Effect of glucocorticoid therapy. *American Journal of Respiratory Cellular and Molecular Biology* 12(5):567-578, 1995.

169. Zwilling BS, Brown D, Pearl D. Induction of major histocompatibility complex class II glycoproteins by interferon-gamma: Attenuation of the effects of restraint stress. *Journal of Neuroimmunology* 37(1-2): 115-122, 1992.

170. Glaser R, Lafuse WP, Bonneau RH, Atkinson C, Kiecolt-Glaser JK. Stress-associated modulation of proto-oncogene expression in human peripheral blood leukocytes. *Behavioral Neurosciences* 107(3):525-529, 1993.

171. Brown DH, Sheridan J, Pearl D, Zwilling BS. Regulation of mycobacterial growth by the hypothalamus-pituitary-adrenal axis: Differential responses of *Mycobacterium bovis*-BCG-resistant and -susceptible mice. *Infection and Immunity* 61(11):4793-4800, 1993.

172. Adler HE, Adler LL, Tobach E. Past, present and future of competitive psychology. *Annals of the New York Academy of Sciences* 223:184-192, 1973.

173. Rook GA, Hernandez-Pando R. The pathogenesis of tuberculosis. *Annual Reviews of Microbiology* 50:259-284, 1996.

174. Rook GA, Stanford JL. The Koch phenomenon and the immunopathology of tuberculosis. *Current Topics in Microbiology and Immunology* 215:239-262, 1996.

175. Raven PW, Checkley SA, Taylor NF. Extra-adrenal effects of metyrapone include inhibition of the 11-oxoreductase activity of 11 beta-hydroxysteroid dehydrogenase: A model for 11-HSD I deficiency. *Clinical Endocrinology* 43(5):637-644, 1995.

176. Raven PW, O'Dwyer AM, Taylor NF, Checkley SA. The relationship between the effects of metyrapone treatment on depressed mood and urinary steroid profiles. *Psychoneuroendocrinology* 21(3):277-286, 1996.

177. Holsboer F, Von Bardeleben U, Gerken A, Stalla GK, Muller OA. Blunted corticotropin and normal cortisol response to human corticotropin-releasing factor in depression. *New England Journal of Medicine* 311(17):1127-1135, 1984.

178. Rupprecht R, Hauser CA, Trapp TA, Holsboer F. Neurosteroids: Molecular mechanisms of action and psychopharmacological significance. *Journal of Steroid Biochemistry and Molecular Biology* 56(1-6):163-168, 1996.

179. Casale GP, Vennerstrom JL, Bavari S, Wang TL. Inhibition of interleukin 2 driven proliferation of mouse CTLL2 cells, by selected carbamate and organophosphate insectivides and congeners of carbaryl. *Immunopharmacology and Immunotoxicology* 15(2-3):199-215, 1993.

180. Suhadolnik RJ, Peterson DL, Cheney PR, Horvath SE, Reichenbach NL, O'Brien K, Lombardi V, Welsh S, Furr EG, Charubala R, Pfleiderer W. Biochemical dysregulation of the 2-5A synthetase/RNase L antiviral defense pathway in chronic fatigue syndrome. *Journal of Chronic Fatigue Syndrome* 5(3/4):223-242, 1999.

181. Vojdani A, Lapp CW. The relationship between chronic fatigue syndrome and chemical exposure. *Journal of Cronic Fatigue Syndrome* 5(3/4):207-221, 1999.

182. Lengyel P. Biochemistry of interferons and their actions. *Annual Review of Biochemistry* 51:251-282, 1982.

183. Sen GC, Ransohoff RM. Interferon-induced antiviral actions and their regulation. *Advances in Virus Research* 42:57-102, 1993.

184. Player MR, Torrence PF. The 2-5A system: Modulation of viral and cellular processes through acceleration of RNA degradation. *Pharmacological Therapy* 78:55-113, 1998.

185. Wells V, Mallucci L. Expression of the 2-5A system during the cell cycle. *Experimental Cell Research* 159:27-36, 1985.

186. Suhadolnik RJ, Reichenbach NL, Hitzges P, Sobol RW, Peterson DL, Henry B, Ablashi DV, Muller WE, Schroder HC, Carter WA, et al. Upregulation of the 2-5A synthetase/RNase L antiviral pathway associated with chronic fatigue syndrome. *Clinical Infectious Diseases* 18:S96-S104, 1994.

187. Suhadolnik RJ, Reichenbach NL, Hitzges P, Adelson ME, Peterson DL, Cheney P, Salvato P, Thompson C, Loveless M, Muller WE, et al. Changes in the 2-5A synthetase/RNase L antiviral pathway in a controlled clinical trial with poly(I)-poly(C_{12}U) in chronic fatigue syndrome. *In Vivo* 8(4):599-604, 1994.

188. Suhadolnik RJ, Peterson DL, O'Brien K, Cheney PR, Herst CV, Reichenbach NL, Kon N, Horrath SE, Iacono KT, Adelson ME, De Meirleir K, De Becker P, Charubala R, Pfeiderer W. Biochemical evidence for a novel low molecular weight 2-5A-dependent RNase L in chronic fatigue syndrome. *Journal of Interferon and Cytokine Research* 17(7):377-385, 1997.

189. Solomon V, Leckert SH, Goldberg AL. The N-end rule pathway catalyzes a major fraction of the protein degradation in skeletal muscle. *Journal of Biological Chemistry* 273:25216-25222, 1998.

190. Borish L, Schmaling K, DiClementi JD, Streib J, Negri J, Jones JF. Chronic fatigue syndrome: Identification of distinct subgroups on the basis of allergy and psychologic variables. *Journal of Allergy and Clinical Immunology* 102(2):222-230, 1998.

191. Patarca R, Lugtendorf S, Antoni M, Klimas NG, Flecther MA. Dysreulated expression of tumor necrosis factor in the chronic fatigue immune dysfunction syndrome: Interrelations with cellular sources and patterns of soluble immune mediator expression. *Clinical Infectious Diseases* 18:S147-S153, 1994.

192. Patarca R, Klimas N, Sandler D, Garcia MN, Fletcher MA. Interindividual immune status variation patterns in patients with chronic fatigue syndrome: Association with the tumor necrosis factor system and gender. *Journal of Chronic Fatigue Syndrome* 2(1):13-19, 1995.

193. Chao CC, Janof EN, Hu SX, Thomas K, Gallagher M, Tsang M, Peterson PK. Altered cytokine release in peripheral blood mononuclear cell cultures from patients with chronic fatigue syndrome. *Cytokine* 3(4):292-298, 1991.

194. Chapekar MS, Glazer RI. The synergistic cytocidal effect produced by immune interferon and tumor necrosis factor in HT-29 cells is associated with inhibition of rRNA processing and (2,5)-oligo(A) activation of RNase L. *Biochemical and Biophysicial Research Communications* 151:1180-1187, 1988.

195. Lieberman PM. Influenza virus vaccine and Epstein-Barr virus infection. *Clincial Ecology* 7(3):51, 1990.

196. Lijima H, Sun S, Cyong JC, Jyonouchi H. Juzen-taiho-to, a Japanese herbal medicine, modulates type 1 and type 2 T-cell responses in old BALB/c mice. *American Journal of Chinese Medicine* 27(2):191-203, 1999.

197. Klimas NG, Fletcher MA. Alteration of type 1/type 2 cytokine pattern following adoptive immunotherapy of patients with chronic fatigue syndrome (CFS) using autologous ex vivo expanded lymph node cells. Abstract, II International Conf. CFS, Brussels, 1999.

198. Klimas NG. Clinical impact of adoptive therapy with purified CD8 cells in HIV infection. *Seminars in Hematology* 29:40-43, 1992.

199. Klimas NG, Fletcher MA, Walling J, Garcia-Morales R, Patarca R, Moody D, Okarma T. Ex vivo CD8 lymphocyte activation, expansion and reinfusion into donors with rIL-2—A phase I study. In *Septieme Colloque des Cent Gardes: Retroviruses of Human AIDS and Related Animal Disease,* M. Girard and L. Valette, Eds., 285-290, 1993.

200. Klimas NG, Patarca R, Walling J, Garcia R, Mayer V, Albarracin C, Moody D, Okarma T, Fletcher MA. Changes in the clinical and immunological stati of AIDS patients upon adoptive therapy with activated autologous CD8+ T cells and interleukin-2 infusion. *Journal of Acquired Immunodeficiency Syndromes* 8:1073-1081, 1994.

201. Klimas NG, Patarca R, Maher K, Smith M, Jin X-Q, Huang H-S, Walling J, Gamber C, Fletcher MA. Immunomodulation with autologous, ex vivo manipulated cytotoxic T lymphocytes in HIV-1 disease. *Clinical Immunology Newsletter* 14:101-105, 1994.

202. Patarca R, Klimas NG, Walling J, Mayer V, Baum M, Yue X-S, Garcia MN, Pons H, Sandler D, Friedlander A, Page B, Lai S, Fletcher MA. CD8 T-cell immunotherapy in AIDFS: Rationale and lessons learned at the cellular and molecular biology levels. *Clinical Immunology Newsletter* 14:105-111, 1994.

203. Patarca R, Klimas NG, Walling J, Sandler D, Friedlander A, Jin X-Q, Garcia MN, Fletcher MA. Adoptive CD8+ T-cell immunotherapy of AIDS patients with Kaposi's sarcoma. *Critical Reviews in Oncogenesis* 6(3-6):179-234, 1995.

204. See DM, Broumand N, Sahl L, Tilles TG. In vitro effects of echinacea and ginseng on natural killer and antibody-dependent cell cytotoxicity in healthy subjects and chronic fatigue syndrome or acquired immunodeficiency syndrome patients. *Immunopharmacology* 35(3):229-235, 1997.

205. Song Z, Kharazmi A, Wu H, Faber V, Moser C, Krogh HK, Rygaard J, Hoiby N. Effects of ginseng treatment on neutrophil chemiluminescence and immunoglobulin G subclasses in a rat model of chronic *Pseudomonas*

aeruginosa pneumonia. *Clinical Diagnostics and Laboratory Immunology* 5(6):882-887, 1998.

206. Cupp MJ. Herbal remedies: Adverse effects and drug interactions. *American Family Physician* 59(5):1239-1245, 1999.

207. Miller LG. Herbal medicinals: Selected clinical considerations focusing on known or potential drug-herb interactions. *Archives of Internal Medicine* 158(20):2200-2211, 1998.

208. McRae S. Elevated serum digoxin levels in a patient taking digoxin and Siberian ginseng. *CMAJ* 155(3):293-295, comment 115(9):1237, 1996.

209. Awang DVC. Siberian ginseng toxicity may be case of mistaken identity. *CMAJ* 155:1237, 1996.

210. Wong HCG. Probable false authentication of herbal plants: Ginseng. *Archives of Internal Medicine* 159:1142, 1999.

211. Rettig MB, Ma HJ, Vescio RA, Pold M, Schiller G, Belson D, Savage A, Nishikubo C, Wu C, Fraser I, Said JW, Berenson JR. Kaposi-sarcoma associated herpesvirus infection of bone marrow dendritic cells from multiple myeloma patients. *Science* 276(5320):1851-1854, 1997.

212. Said JW, Rettig MR, Heppner K, Vescio RA, Schiller G, Ma HJ, Belson D, Savage A, Shintaku IP, Koeffler HP, Asou H, Pinkus G, Pinkus J, Schrage M, Green E, Berenson JR. Localization of Kaposi's sarcoma-associated herpesvirus in bone marrow biopsy samples from patients with multiple myeloma. *Blood* 90(11), 4278-4282, 1997.

213. DeGreef C, Van DeVoorde W, Bakkus M, Corthals J, Heirman C, Schots R, Lacor P, Van Camp B, Van Riet I. Kaposi's sarcoma-associated herpesvirus (KSHV/HHV-8) DNA sequences are absent in lieukapheresis products and ex vivo expanded CD34+ cells from multiple myeloma patients. *British Journal of Haematology* 106(4): 1033-1036, 1999.

214. Levine PH. The use of transfer factors in chronic fatigue syndrome: Prospects and problems. *Biotherapy* 9(1-3):77-79, 1996.

215. Ablashi DV, Levine PH, De Vinci C, Whitman JE Jr, Pizza G, Viza D. The use of anti HHV-6 transfer factor for the treatment of two patients with chronic fatigue syndrome (CFS). Two case reports. *Biotherapy* 1996; 9(1-3):81-86, 1996.

216. De Vinci C, Levine PH, Pizza G, Fudenberg HH, Orens P, Pearson G, Viza D. Lessons from a pilot study of transfer factor in chronic fatigue syndrome. *Biotherapy* 9(1-3):87-90, 1996.

217. Hana I, Vrubel J, Pekarek J, Cech K. The influence of age on transfer factor treatment of cellular immunodeficiency, chronic fatigue syndrome and/or chronic viral infections. *Biotherapy* 9(1-3):91-95, 1996.

Index

Order Your Own Copy of
This Important Book for Your Personal Library!

TREATMENT OF CHRONIC FATIGUE SYNDROME IN THE ANTIVIRAL REVOLUTION ERA

_____in hardbound at $34.95 (ISBN: 0-7890-1253-7)

_____in softbound at $19.95 (ISBN: 0-7890-1254-5)

COST OF BOOKS_____

OUTSIDE USA/CANADA/
MEXICO: ADD 20%____

POSTAGE & HANDLING_____
*(US: $4.00 for first book & $1.50
for each additional book)*
*Outside US: $5.00 for first book
& $2.00 for each additional book)*

SUBTOTAL_____

in Canada: add 7% GST____

STATE TAX____
*(NY, OH & MIN residents, please
add appropriate local sales tax)*

FINAL TOTAL____
*(If paying in Canadian funds,
convert using the current
exchange rate, UNESCO
coupons welcome.)*

❑ **BILL ME LATER:** ($5 service charge will be added)
(Bill-me option is good on US/Canada/Mexico orders only;
not good to jobbers, wholesalers, or subscription agencies.)

❑ Check here if billing address is different from
shipping address and attach purchase order and
billing address information.

Signature_____

❑ **PAYMENT ENCLOSED: $_____**

❑ **PLEASE CHARGE TO MY CREDIT CARD.**

❑ Visa ❑ MasterCard ❑ AmEx ❑ Discover
❑ Diner's Club ❑ Eurocard ❑ JCB

Account # _____

Exp. Date_____

Signature_____

Prices in US dollars and subject to change without notice.

NAME_____

INSTITUTION_____

ADDRESS_____

CITY_____

STATE/ZIP_____

COUNTRY_____ COUNTY (NY residents only)_____

TEL_____ FAX_____

E-MAIL_____

May we use your e-mail address for confirmations and other types of information? ❑ Yes ❑ No
We appreciate receiving your e-mail address and fax number. Haworth would like to e-mail or fax special
discount offers to you, as a preferred customer. **We will never share, rent, or exchange your e-mail address
or fax number.** We regard such actions as an invasion of your privacy.

Order From Your Local Bookstore or Directly From
The Haworth Press, Inc.
10 Alice Street, Binghamton, New York 13904-1580 • USA
TELEPHONE: 1-800-HAWORTH (1-800-429-6784) / Outside US/Canada: (607) 722-5857
FAX: 1-800-895-0582 / Outside US/Canada: (607) 722-6362
E-mail: getinfo@haworthpressinc.com
PLEASE PHOTOCOPY THIS FORM FOR YOUR PERSONAL USE.
www.HaworthPress.com

BOF00